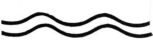

HEAVE HO

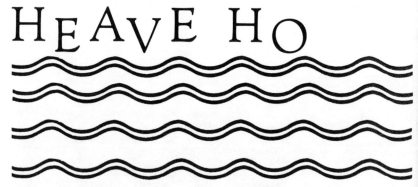

My Little Green Book of Seasickness

by Charles Mazel "et Al."

Illustrations by Polly Jordon

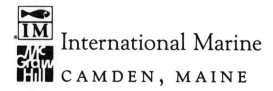

International Marine

CAMDEN, MAINE

Published by International Marine

10 9 8 7 6 5 4 3 2

Copyright © 1992 International Marine, an imprint of
TAB Books. TAB Books is a division of McGraw-Hill,
Inc.

Library of Congress Cataloging-in-Publication Data
Mazel, Charles.
    Heave ho : my little green book of seasickness / Charles Mazel.
        p.   cm.
    Includes index.
    ISBN 0-87742-324-5
    1. Motion sickness—Humor. 2. Motion sickness—Miscellanea.
I. Title.
RC103.M6M39   1992
616.9'892—dc20   92-11119
                                                            CIP

Questions regarding the content of this book should be addressed to:
        International Marine
        P.O. Box 220
        Camden, ME 04843

Text design by James Brisson.
Text composition by A&B Typesetters, Bow, New Hampshire.

CONTENTS

ACKNOWLEDGMENTS

This book was written by Charlie Mazel "et Al." For those who know their Latin abbreviations, this is no mistake. A real Al, Albert Franchi, M.D., earns special notice for his role as collaborator, idea bouncer and bouncee, and general associate in charge of lunacy.

The "et al." are the many others who deserve credit and thanks:

The authors whose writings I have pillaged;

Polly Jordan, for her translation of words into pictures;

Jim Babb, editor de luxe;

Chuck Oman, for his valuable advice;

Family and friends who offered constructive criticism on early drafts;

Walter Lee Eddins, for his story and sense of humor;

The Isabella Stewart Gardner Museum in Boston;

Manuscript Collection, G.W. Blunt White Library, Mystic Seaport Museum, Mystic, Connecticut;

Libraries in general, and the research section of the Boston Public Library in particular;

Schoenhof's Foreign Books in Harvard Square;

The Lancet, a treasure trove of medical history;

My wife, Ellen, for her unfailing support and contribution of good ideas, and my daughters, Lauren and Charlotte;

And last but far from least, the sea – which I love well enough to share my meals with.

FOREWORD

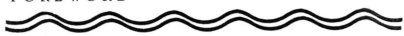

Charles M. Oman

When did you first feel motion sick?

For many of us, the question immediately evokes an unpleasant childhood memory. Perhaps we can recall a sudden roadside stop during a family auto trip, or the embarrassing aftermath of a whirling carnival ride. As adults, we usually are a little less susceptible, but when we do experience an attack of frank seasickness, carsickness, or airsickness, we still feel intense nausea and profound embarrassment. Fortunately, for many people this doesn't happen often. Airliners today fly high in smooth air, and cruise ships are equipped with stabilizers. But when we are exposed to unusual motion—perhaps traveling in a commuter plane, or driving on a winding mountain road, or sailing the open ocean—we are reminded of our intrinsic gastric frailty. As-

Charles M. Oman, Ph.D., is director of the Man-Vehicle Laboratory in the Department of Aeronautics and Astronautics at Massachusetts Institute of Technology. He is an authority on inner ear balance function and motion sickness. His research has included major experiments on four NASA Spacelab missions. A lifelong sailor, Chuck has done five Newport-Bermuda races, and has written for SAIL and Cruising World magazines.

tronauts are no exception. Many are test pilots and not susceptible to airsickness, but in space two-thirds of them experience
symptoms. Their well-publicized problems over the past decade
have led to extensive research on motion sickness, from which a
good deal has been learned. Judiciously chosen drugs can raise
your threshold for feeling ill. In any given situation, there usually
are things you can do to reduce the stimulus. We know that motion sickness results when "sensory conflict" signals in the brain's
balance and posture control centers somehow spill over to
nearby centers that trigger vomiting. Unfortunately, the physiol-
ogy of the linkage still hasn't been worked out and, as yet, there
are still no magic cures.

Charlie Mazel is an avid sailor and scuba diver and widely
traveled ocean engineer and marine biologist. I am also a sailor,
and my own research at MIT is on spatial disorientation, inner
ear function, and motion sickness. When Charlie and I first met
and started swapping stories a couple of years ago, we soon discovered that we shared the misfortune of being both vocation-
ally and avocationally afflicted. Charlie says he likes going to sea
far more than he dislikes his occasional bouts with seasickness.
I've always thought that if you're a sailor who's never been seasick, you probably just haven't sailed enough. Charlie shares my
belief that motion sickness isn't really a "sickness" at all, but just
a normal human response to abnormal motion. Once you get
over the embarrassment of feeling bad, it is amazing how much
better you feel. Undoubtedly the best way to do this is with
laughter. Charlie's purpose in writing this book is to remind us
that there is much to laugh about.

Charlie's book is a wonderful, lighthearted anthology of the
older seasickness literature—with some of his own limericks
mixed in to flavor the soup. You'll hear from many noted suscep-
tibles, including Seneca and Cicero, Byron, Bessemer and
Barnum, Nelson, Darwin, and Twain. Many lesser known but
well-intentioned physicians offer advice—all of it colorful—and
much of it contradictory. Anti-seasickness belts, electrical stimu-
lators, potions of all kinds. Advice on etiquette, and how to say
"I'm seasick" in 51 languages—a Bartlett's Quotations–like seasickness potpourri. If you suffer frequently from motion sickness,
there is a great deal here worth knowing. Not just because it is
funny, but because it is important to know how to distinguish

between nostrums, placebos, and the truly effective cures. Charlie also offers some serious advice on seasickness prevention and treatment, based on present-day scientific knowledge. This is not a medical book, but it is one that will amuse and enlighten every person who travels, works, or plays on the ocean.

INTRODUCTION

Seasickness. The very word turns the stomach, turns the cheeks a bilious shade of green, and turns honest people into liars ("Who, me? Never!"). According to surveys it is the number one reason most people give for not vacationing on a cruise ship.

But is seasickness really such a threat? Consider the lesson learned by P.T. Barnum, the Greatest Showman on Earth. In 1844 he crossed the Atlantic to exhibit General Tom Thumb to the crowned heads of Europe.

> *For the benefit of "land lubbers" who fear to go out of sight of land, I will mention that I had all my life been desirous of visiting Europe; but the terrible fear which I had of the Atlantic, and the dread of sea-sickness, of which I had heard so many horrid accounts, hitherto deterred me. I found, however, on trying it, that "the devil is never so black as he is painted"; for on neither occasion was I sick for a moment, nor were more than one in ten of the passengers. To some, no doubt, the sea is exceedingly unpleasant, on account of sickness; but generally it lasts but a few days—frequently it does not occur at all, and, on the whole, it is a mere bug-bear, calculated to frighten timid persons out of the idea of leaving home.*
>
> —P.T. BARNUM, *NEW YORK ATLAS*, 1844

Barnum was writing at a time when the cause of seasickness was still unknown, and there were as many home remedies as there were people who had been seasick. The affliction has been with us for thousands of years, but it's only within the last fifty that we've really begun to gain an understanding of its causes, prevention, and treatment.

Many, many people, including this author, have been going to sea for years and leaving a part of themselves behind, returning only with their sense of humor. Seasickness can be funny—especially for those who aren't suffering. Through the ages there have been unending attempts to explain the disease and to combat it through potions, diets, muscular regimens, mechanical devices, and sheer willpower. This compendium of facts and fictions, nostrums and notions, preventives and prevarications, readings and reflections concerning the bane of sea-travelers is dedicated to all my fellow sufferers.

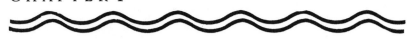

CHAPTER I

WHY THIS QUALMISH, WHENCE THIS QUEASY MOOD? *The Unnatural Nature of Mal de Mer*

Perhaps no malady to which mankind is subject is productive of so much real suffering, with so low a percentage of mortality, as the peculiar affliction known as seasickness.

— *SCIENTIFIC AMERICAN*, 1912

WHAT is seasickness?

Homesickness is a longing to be at home. Seasickness is not a longing to be at sea. Nor does it mean you're fed up with being at sea, any more than being morning sick means you're fed up with mornings. The poet makes a clear distinction between the two:

I have been seasick, and sick of the sea.
— LORD BYRON, 1809, IN A LETTER TO A FRIEND

Seasickness really is a sickness, suddenly striking perfectly healthy people in almost any kind of weather and departing just as quickly as it arrived. Unlike most ailments, seasickness is self-inflicted: If you don't go to sea, you don't get it. It isn't carried by germs, so it isn't contagious by contact, yet any sufferer can tell you that it is psychologically contagious in the extreme. The sight of a stranger in its grip, an odor, or even a memory, can trigger an attack.

Seasickness, as we shall see, is just one form of motion sickness.

Motion sickness is unique among all the illnesses that afflict man. In common with childbirth (which is not normally con-

3

sidered an illness), it can cause complete temporary incapacita-
tion without any pathological basis and entirely by reflex
mechanisms, though unlike childbirth it serves no obvious
purpose at all.

— GLASER, PROCEEDINGS OF THE ROYAL SOCIETY OF
MEDICINE, 1959

HOW do you know when you're seasick?

A stout wooden wedge driven in at my right temple and out
at my left, a floating deposit of lukewarm oil in my throat,
and a compression of the bridge of my nose in a blunt pair of
pincers, these are the personal sensations by which I know we
are off.

— CHARLES DICKENS, *THE CALAIS NIGHT-MAIL*, 1861

Seasickness manifests itself in many forms, from a vague feeling of dislocation to an imperious notice to your last meal to
evacuate the premises immediately. According to researchers in
the field, The Big Four Symptoms are:

- **Pallor:** White or whitish-greenish skin, for which there is
  no counterpart in the 64-pack of Crayolas.

- **Cold sweats:** Like the feeling you get trying to convince
  Sister Mary Eunice that your dog ate your homework.

- **Nausea:** The Ancient Greeks understood the intimate re-
  lationship between going to sea and losing your lunch. It's
  only a short skip to the rail from *ναυσ* (naus) — their word
  for ship — to nausea.

- **Vomiting:** The biggest of The Big Four. You can hide or
  explain away all the other symptoms, but there's no deny-
  ing this one.

In addition to The Big Four, here are some popular auxiliary
symptoms:

dry lips	headache	drowsiness	dizziness
salivation	yawning	belching	flatulence

Look around you: Is your fishing buddy seasick? Or did he just have beans for breakfast?

Researchers also mention impaired mental activity as a consequence of *mal de mer*:

> Many of the greatest minds of the world have been upon the ocean, but how few great thoughts have been conceived at sea. Men of the highest genius seem to be transformed as soon as they get at a distance from land in a rolling ship.
> —GEORGE M. BEARD, M.D., *PRACTICAL TREATISE ON SEASICKNESS*, 1880

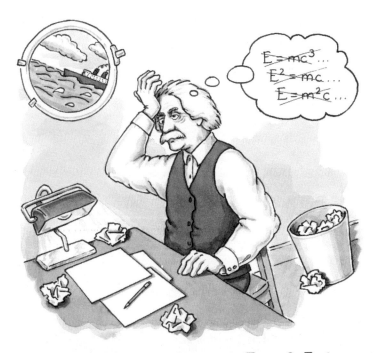

EINSTEIN AT SEA

A poet bespied a bright comet,
And commenced to composing a sonnet.
As he searched for a rhyme,
The waves they did climb,
Now all he can think of is . . . vomit.

Another popular symptom of seasickness is <u>soporific lassi-tude,</u> a complete collapse into inactivity and a total disregard for your surroundings.

> *I saw a man once, a courageous talker, urging his crew to sail in threatening weather. At sea, with the storm raging, you would find him without a word to say, under his cloak, for anyone to trample on who chose to.*
>
> —SOPHOCLES, *AJAX*, CIRCA 450 BC

This malaise was taken for granted in ancient times. Plato even used it as an analogy to explain what might happen when one is confronted with false arguments:

> *If we are completely baffled, then I suppose we must be humble and let the argument do with us what it will, like a sailor trampling over seasick passengers.*
>
> —PLATO, *THEAETETUS* 191A, 4TH CENTURY BC
> (CORNFORD TRANSLATION, 1957)

Anacharsis, a Greek philosopher of the 6th century BC, was once asked, "Which are there more of, the living or the dead?" Anacharsis asked in return, "In which group should I count those who are sailing on the sea?"

The seasick hover in a state somewhere between life and death, not caring in which direction fate takes them. They are suspended in a state of purge-atory.

WHAT does it really feel like to be seasick?

> *But why this qualmish, whence this queasy mood?*
> *Have I swill'd flagons? swallowed noisome food?*
> *Drugs I abhor, nor have I lately fed*
> *With foreign beaux, who cleanse their plates with bread;*
> *Nor native boors, who pick—beyond belief—*
> *Their tusks with forks, then stick them in their beef:*
> *No mental loathings float upon the brain,*
> *No dire prognosis from a tribe insane,*
> *Disease the fancy—yet—slow languors creep,*

(continued on page 8)

PURGE - ATORY

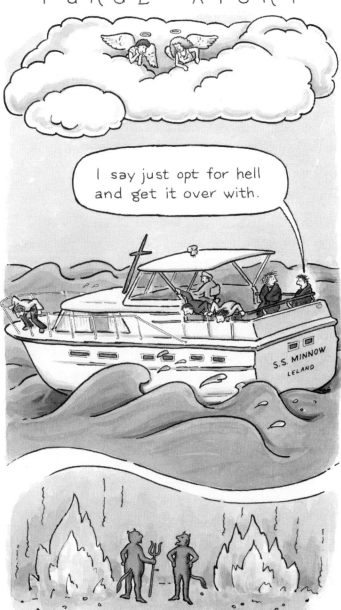

Contagion low'rs — chill dews the temples steep,
Man's proud pre-eminence expiring lies,
And the last banquet — soon — too soon will rise.

Dear, rich repast, the call of Nature wait,
Let her conduct thee to the postern gate,
There unreprov'd and hid from vulgar eyes,
Indulge the luxury of parting sighs!
O! hand a vase — alas! alas! — too late —
Weep, weep controllers of the bed of state —
Some healing hand for pity hold my brows —
Seraphic pens, record spontaneous vows!
If once on shore — away — a sluice prevails,
The world is delug'd! — sponges, mops, and pails!
— "THE SEA-SICK MINSTREL OR MARITIME SORROWS"
ANONYMOUS, LONDON 1796

HOW does it strike?

Once seasickness begins, it advances quickly. Researchers call this the *avalanche phenomenon.* Just a small push can trigger a slide, which builds in volume and velocity as it thunders along its inexorable course.

> The attack begins as a rule with yawning or sighing; sooner or later there is nausea; and the last straw is supplied by the smell of a cigar or the careless remark of a bystander.
> — BENNETT, *BRITISH MEDICAL JOURNAL*, 1928

The avalanche phenomenon often leads to another natural disaster, the *volcano phenomenon:* a sudden and violent eruption of your meals *du jour.*

> There once was a man from Nantucket
> Who at sea always carried a bucket.
> When he was asked why,
> He replied with a sigh,
> "I never know when I'll upchuck it."

WHERE do you get seasick?

At sea, of course.

Plenty of people throughout history recognized this and therefore had no use for the sea—and didn't hesitate to say so:

> *Marcus Cato said that he had never repented but three times in his whole life, once was when he paid a ship's fare to a place instead of walking.*
>
> — PLUTARCH, CIRCA 110 AD

> *If you can get there by land, do not go by water.*
>
> — CHINESE PROVERB

> *A man who goes to sea for pleasure would go to hell for a pastime.*
>
> — SAMUEL JOHNSON

> *I never saw the use of the sea. Many a sad heart it has caused, and many a sick stomach has it occasioned.*
>
> — BENJAMIN DISRAELI

> *For the sea is as nonsensical a thing as any going. It never knows what to do with itself. It hasn't got no employment for its mind, and is always in a state of vacancy. Like them polar bears in the wild-beast shows as is constantly a-nodding their heads from side to side, it never can be quiet. Which is entirely owing to its uncommon stupidity.*
>
> — CHARLES DICKENS, *MARTIN CHUZZLEWIT*, 1843

Some seasick-prone people like to go to sea anyway, and may even make it a central part of their lives. W.I.B. Crealock, the famous long-distance sailor and sailboat designer, said:

> *Providence, while granting me an intense love of the sea, unfortunately failed to provide me with an interior suitable for its enjoyment, and I was usually among the first to make my little offering to the deep.*
>
> — W.I.B. CREALOCK, *VAGABONDING UNDER SAIL*, 1951

WHAT kinds of motion bring on seasickness?

It is not during the storm, when mountain waves lift the prow of the vessel now high in the air, and now plunge it as though it were steered for the ocean's bed, that sea-sickness most prevails. It is the chopping sea after the storm that conquers the stomach of even the weather-worn sea-farer. . . . The unenviable notoriety of the English Channel, as a region where the stoutest knees tremble and the ruddiest faces grow pale, arises not from any superiority in the height of waves, but from their unequal character.

— STEVENS, *SCRIBNER'S MONTHLY,* JULY 1883

Some people are just more seasick-prone than others, but there are additional factors at work. An obvious one is the strength of the motions, but just as important is how frequently they occur. Scientific experiments have shown that ship motions repeated at a rate of once every three seconds to once every 10 seconds are the most effective at producing queasiness (in technical terms, the most *nauseogenic*). If the same strength of motion occurs at a much faster or slower rate it is less likely to produce seasickness. Unfortunately for sea travelers, this "worst" frequency corresponds exactly with the usual frequency range for waves at sea.

WHERE did seasickness come from?

When the first multicellular organism crawled from the sea, the sudden absence of motion was too much to bear: it promptly threw up all over the sand. It was so sick it couldn't even crawl back into the water, and from that ancient ancestor humans evolved. Except for an occasional dip in the neighbor's gene pool, all of that evolution occurred on land. Somewhere along the way, humans lost any remaining ancestral affinity for ocean travel.

The human nervous system still remains that of a self-propelled animal designed to move at foot-pace through an

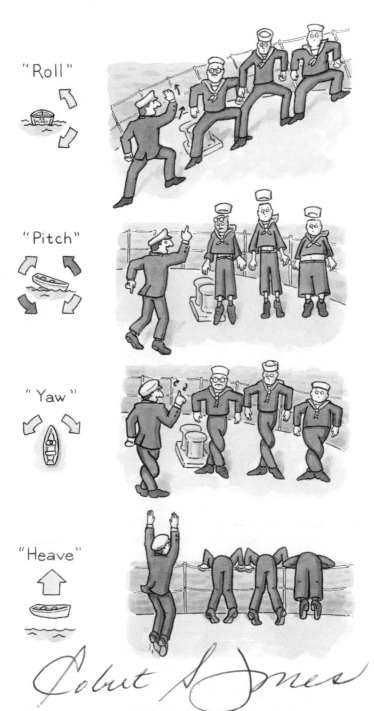

"Roll"

"Pitch"

"Yaw"

"Heave"

essentially two-dimensional environment under normal
earth gravity.
— REASON & BRAND, *MOTION SICKNESS,* 1975

"But," you may ask, "humans have been going to sea ever since the first Neanderthal sneaked out on a log to go bass fishing. Why haven't we evolved a resistance to seasickness?"

Unfortunately, human evolution is slow. To evolution, thousands of years is just a coffee break. But if humans have been slow to evolve, seasickness has readily adapted itself to the latest trends in travel. Arab traders were stricken while voyaging on the ships of the desert, Indian maharajahs while riding elephants, travelers in the early west on stagecoaches. Today, people routinely become sick on cars, buses, trains, and roller coasters, usually in the seat next to you.

Riders borne by human carriers in sedan chairs or on litters
can also experience motion sickness, particularly when carried
in stately procession by several bearers striding in unison. At
least one pontiff in recent times is reputed to have been nause-
ated by the motion of the papal seda.
— GUIGNARD AND MCCAULEY, "THE ACCELERATIVE
STIMULUS FOR MOTION SICKNESS," IN
MOTION AND SPACE SICKNESS,
G. H. CRAMPTON (ED.), 1990

Seasickness has followed us off the earth and into the sky, to become airsickness. It has even relentlessly pursued us into the heavens and taken up residence as space sickness, one of the main problems facing astronauts:

"What happened?" whispered Arthur in considerable awe.
"We took off," said Slartibartfast.
Arthur lay in startled stillness on the acceleration couch. He
wasn't certain whether he had just got space-sickness or reli-
gion.
— DOUGLAS ADAMS, *LIFE, THE UNIVERSE, AND*
EVERYTHING, 1982

As yet there are no data to indicate whether time sickness will be waiting for us when we voyage into the fourth dimension, and whether time travelers will become sick before, during, or after their trip.

WHY is there seasickness?

According to some recent scientific thinking, the physiological mechanisms that bring on the urge to purge do serve an evolutionary function: They protect us from being poisoned. Our body lets us know we've ingested something bad (like the shrimp salad the hostess swore was OK, or the better part of a bottle of Usher's Green Stripe) when we become dizzy. The brain receives that signal and informs the stomach, which unceremoniously shows the offending party the door.

The sea's motion acts on the vestibular system in our inner ear, in effect producing the same signals in our brain as are produced by some poisons. People with damaged vestibular systems don't get seasick. (Chronic sufferers may wish to experiment by exploring their ears with any object larger than their elbows.)

One leading researcher draws an analogy between motion sickness and the knee-jerk response. Evolution did not design your leg to shoot out at the tap of a rubber hammer; reflexes simply keep your leg stable in normal use. It's purely coincidental that when you tap that spot just so, out goes the leg. Similarly, when you go out to sea, out goes the lunch.

IS seasickness good for anything?

Perhaps. Through the ages, some doctors felt that a period of purging the system through seasickness would be therapeutic.

> *Sea-sickness is a very unpleasant but often a very beneficial occurrence, and in many cases might with more propriety be sought than avoided. It may not unfrequently be regarded as an excellent preliminary to a residence at the watering place which is the destination of the voyager.*
> — ANONYMOUS, *THE LANCET*, 1832

In the age of medicine that brought us medicinal bleeding and night vapors, doctors often sent patients on voyages for the sole

purpose of inducing vomiting. One doctor prescribed just such a
course for a stubborn case of jaundice:

> *I one day, when the sea was rough, recommended her sailing
> in a boat for three or four hours; she at once followed the
> advice, and to use her own words, was horribly sick. The
> patient was cured at once by it, and where it is not so immedi-
> ately beneficial (as will most probably generally be the case) it
> might be persevered in, with intervals of a few days, with a
> reasonable prospect of success.*
>
> —DR. PERCY, *THE LANCET*, 1844

Even in the days before TV advertising made self-diagnosis a
universal passion, individuals might prescribe a vomiting voyage
for themselves:

> *I once met a literary gentleman, who, on a voyage across the
> Northern Atlantic, tried every means to make himself sea-sick,
> in order that he might get the benefit of the trip, and failed,
> and was utterly disappointed. He smoked strong cigars in great
> excess, exposed himself in every way, and sought eagerly the
> symptoms that most people dread and flee from.*
>
> —GEORGE M. BEARD, *A PRACTICAL TREATISE ON
> SEA-SICKNESS*, 1880

Dr. Beard did not share this attitude himself, for he went on
to write, "There is, on scientific grounds, no more reason for
seeking an attack of sea-sickness than for seeking an attack of ty-
phoid fever."

The unpleasant effects of motion sickness have even been
used as a tool for behavior modification. In 1843 a German author described

> *a device which resembled a small sentry-box and was sus-
> pended on pivots outside the Town Hall, and was commonly
> used as a punishment for delinquent youths. The offender was
> placed inside and the box was rotated very rapidly by a police-
> man until the offender had given a "disgusting spectacle" to the
> onlookers.*
>
> —QUOTED IN REASON & BRAND, *MOTION
> SICKNESS*, 1975

No matter where you stand on seasickness—pro or con—you might as well have a good attitude about it.

> *Many persons will tell you that it is an excellent thing to be sea-sick, as you are so much better for it afterwards. If you are a sufferer you will do well to accept their statements as entirely correct, since you are thereby consoled and soothed, and the malady doesn't care what you think about it, one way or the other.*
>
> —THOMAS W. KNOX, *HOW TO TRAVEL*, 1897

For there are no situations, no matter how it may seem at the time, that are entirely without advantage.

> *Seasickness has its obvious disadvantages but it is a wonderful training for sprinters. I have seen old gentlemen with gout disdain their crutches when the Urge came, and make the rail in nothing flat.*
>
> —BASIL WOON, *THE FRANTIC ATLANTIC*, 1927

Seasickness is perhaps unequaled as a regimen for weight loss, a topic we will explore further in Chapter 6.

WHO gets seasick?

> *"And I'm never, never sick at sea."*
> *"What, never?"*
> *"No, never!"*
> *"What, never?"*
> *"Well, hardly ever."*
>
> —GILBERT & SULLIVAN, *HMS PINAFORE*, 1878

Almost no one *never* gets seasick. There's even a standing bet in serious motion sickness laboratories that anyone with an intact vestibular system can be made a victim, given sufficient stimuli. Still, there have been many attempts to categorize people into susceptible and immune groups, among them:

> *Thinkers, brain-workers, women, and the sick and nervous, the fearful, and members of the Latin race, are more suscepti-*

ble than young children, the very old and weak, deaf, drunk,
blind, deafmutes, and members of the Anglo-Saxon race who
are more or less of a phlegmatic temperament. Babies, persons
of high courage and in good physical condition, such as acrobats or athletes, are immune, or less affected, from seasickness.
The same is true of newly acquainted lovers. I found them
always too busy to be bothered with seasickness.

—CAPT. VICTOR SEIDELHUBER, *NO MORE
SEASICKNESS*, 1935

The relatively immune to naupathia are: those with high
blood pressure, the feverish, the deaf and dumb, tabetics
[syphilitics], rope walkers, acrobats, dancers, the insane, and
young children.

—DR. J. BOHEC, PHYSICIAN-IN-CHIEF OF THE *ILE DE
FRANCE*, QUOTED IN TOUBIB, *HYGEIA*, 1937

Americans of both sexes, who are far more nervous than the
English, suffer more from sea-sickness than the English do.

—BEARD, *A PRACTICAL TREATISE ON
SEA-SICKNESS*, 1880

Persons with pendulous and flaccid abdomens suffer as a rule
more intensely from sea-sickness than others.

—NUNN, *THE LANCET*, 1881

At the risk of repeating this *ad nauseam*, seasickness is perfectly natural for almost all of us, no matter how many hours
you've worked out on your Easy Glider.

It is an old adage that there is nothing worse than the sea to
confound a man, be he ever so strong.

—HOMER, CIRCA 800 BC

If we accept the definition of disease as a deviation from the
normal average condition, it follows that liability to seasickness is the normal average condition and not a departure
therefrom. It is a normal response to an abnormal environment. . . . It is as natural for the novice to be sea-sick in
stormy weather as for the toddler to stumble or the inexpert
golfer to foozle his drive.

—HILL, *BRITISH MEDICAL JOURNAL*, 1936

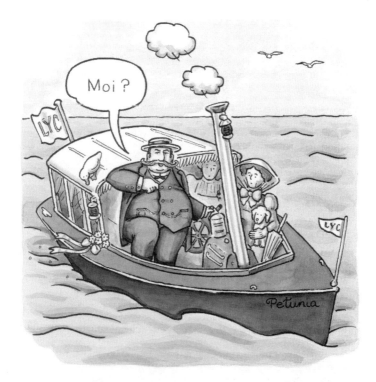

Wide variations in susceptibility to seasickness do exist, however. Some people seem never to become seasick under any conditions, while others succumb at the dock. In the past, researchers believed that women were more susceptible than men, perhaps to atone for their longer lifespans.

> *Females, though a little more inclined to be sick than men, are still very hardy at sea, and probably accommodate themselves more speedily and completely to the circumstances than the other sex. Generally speaking, they can be managed by a little attention, and a few words bordering upon flattery.*
> — ROBERT MUDIE, *THE EMIGRANT'S POCKET COMPANION,* 1832 (TO WHOM JUSTIFIABLY OUTRAGED FEMINISTS SHOULD ADDRESS THEIR LETTER BOMBS)

Age is an important factor, and children are especially susceptible. Perhaps this is the origin of the phrase, "Women and children first."

Seasickness through life:

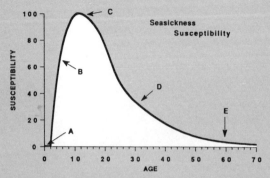

Data for graph from: "Motion sickness susceptibility and behavior," Charles
S. Mirabile Jr., in G. H. Crampton, *Motion and Space Sickness*, 1990

Explanation of graph:

A – The nervous systems of infants and toddlers under the
age of two are not well developed, and they are immune to seasickness. This point is strictly academic, of
course, as members of this age group throw up regu-
larly whether they're moving or not.

B – Susceptibility to motion sickness increases rapidly.
Children of this age may void their stomachs at the
least jostling. They should be kept downwind at all
times.

C – Maximum susceptibility. This does not mean that
everyone goes through the same level of susceptibility – just the same pattern. Some people won't get seasick even at their most susceptible period; others will
remain at C-level for the duration.

D – Your susceptibility to seasickness is decreasing, but so
what? Your kids are on the other side of the curve, and
you're still holding the bucket.

E – Free at Last. The kids are out of the house and you're
ready to enjoy your golden years on the sea. Whether
this means going on a cruise or buying that dream
boat, now you have the time, the money, and the
stomach for it.

Fortunately (or unfortunately, depending on your skill at choosing parents), economic status is not a factor in whether or not you make your sea voyage by rail.

> *What of the poor man? He hires a boat and gets just as sick as the rich man who sails in his yacht.*
> —HORACE, *EPISTLES*, CIRCA 20 BC

Take comfort in knowing that many famous and unlikely people were subject to seasickness. Perhaps the most famous seaman in British naval history, Admiral Horatio Nelson, the hero of Trafalgar, was stricken by seasickness at the start of every voyage. The English admiral and explorer Sir John Franklin, who sought the Northwest Passage, was reputedly "unable to take charge of his ship until it had passed the Bay of Biscay."

And what about the author of these immortal lines?

> *I must go down to the seas again, to the lonely sea and*
> *   the sky,*
> *And all I ask is a tall ship and a star to steer her by.*
> —JOHN MASEFIELD, "SEA FEVER," PUBLISHED IN
> *SALT WATER BALLADS*, 1902

Masefield became known as the "poet of the sea" for verses such as these. But how much "of the sea" was he? As a lad of 13 he shipped out on the *Gilcruix*, but he left the seafaring life soon after due to, what else, severe seasickness.

Some other seasick notables:

Horace, the Roman poet

Charles Darwin

Charles Dickens

Mark Twain

President Woodrow Wilson

General Douglas MacArthur

John James Audubon

Michaelangelo (the turtle, not the artist)

Bluto, arch-enemy of Popeye the Sailor Man

Julius Caesar

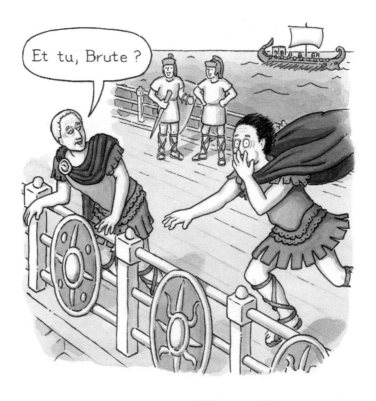

Humans aren't the only creatures subject to seasickness. Chickens, dogs, cats, sheep, cows, monkeys, rats, and horses are all fellow sufferers, as Julius Caesar learned in his military campaign in Africa.

> *Caesar's cavalry found that their horses, worn out with the effects of recent seasickness, were reluctant to keep on the move in pursuit of the enemy.*
>
> —*BELLUM AFRICANUM*, 47 BC

Puppies, rabbits, guinea pigs, and elephants (except for Dr. Seuss's egg-hatching Horton) are reportedly immune. Seasickness is not just confined to land animals, though. The malady has affected seals transported by ship. There's even a report of seasick fish:

> A certain lot of cod, after being kept and handled in the labora-
> tory tanks all one summer, were placed in a tank aboard a boat
> for transportation in the autumn. They had been fed an hour or
> so before being put on the boat. This handling produced no
> effect. However, after the boat had been under way for some
> time, all the feed they had eaten was seen to be on the bottom
> of the tank. Thus, even codfish, after being ashore for some
> time, may become seasick when an ocean voyage is undertaken.
> — MCKENZIE, "CODFISH IN CAPTIVITY," *PROGRESS REPORTS OF
> THE ATLANTIC BIOLOGICAL STATION*, HALIFAX, NS, 1935

We wonder if this variability of seasickness in animals explains why there are no unicorns.

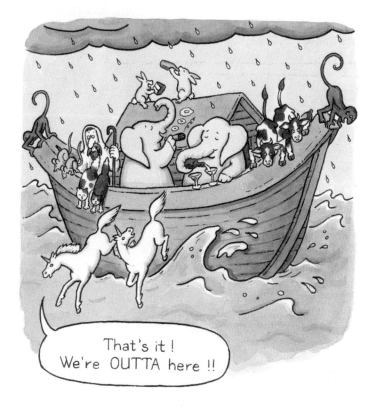

All this theory notwithstanding, there's no foolproof way of determining if you will become seasick. If you got sick riding your tricycle, expect to be sick on the bounding main. If you kept down three chili dogs and a chocolate shake while riding the Cyclone at Coney Island, the lonely sea may be just the place for you. Here's a test you can try in the comfort of your own home:

> Many people have a genuine curiosity to know if they would be seasick in case they should take an ocean voyage. An easy way to put the matter to a test is to stand before the ordinary bureau mirror that turns in its frame, and let some one move it slowly and slightly at first, and gradually growing faster, while you look fixedly at your own reflection. If you feel no effect whatever from it, the chances are that you can stand an ordinary sea voyage without any qualm.
>
> — HOYT, *OLD OCEAN'S FERRY*, 1900

If your decor doesn't run to free-spinning mirrors, here's a short questionnaire to test your sensitivity to seasickness.

Do you get queasy:

looking at your reflection just after you wake up?

paddling an inner tube in a swimming pool?

playing with toy boats in the bathtub?

watching *Mutiny on the Bounty?*

watching fans do "the wave" at sporting events?

watching a bowl of Jello shake?

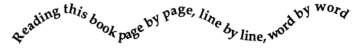

Reading this book page by page, line by line, word by word

CHAPTER 2

THE BOUNCING BRAIN
AND OTHER THEORIES

> *Of all maladies, seasickness must have the record both*
> *for the number of theories as to cause and for the*
> *diversity of methods of treatment. More remarkable are*
> *the facts that most of the theories are right—in part—*
> *and that all the treatments, no matter how ridiculous*
> *they may seem, work—sometimes.*
>
> —ROBERT TOUBIB, "SEASICKNESS," *HYGEIA*, 1937

Possibly the earliest recorded theory about the cause of seasickness dates back some 2,300 years to Hippocrates, The Father of Medicine, who said: "sailing on the sea proves that motion disorders the body." Not very specific, but accurate. It was more than 2,000 years before the term motion sickness was coined. Through history, many people were convinced that seasickness was in fact caused by something special about the sea. Like its smell.

> *Why are people more liable to be seasick when on a sea voyage than on rivers, even though they have calm weather for the voyage?*
> *Are we to say that of all sensations it is smell, and of all emotions fear, that most conduces to sickness? Certainly people tremble and shiver and their bowels turn to water when imagining some danger. But neither of the above causes troubles people who travel by river: everybody's sense of smell is accustomed to fresh water, such as one can drink, and there is no danger in the passage. At sea, on the other hand, men find the smell disagreeable because of its strangeness, and not trusting the present weather to last, are anxious about what the future*

23

holds. *Thus the calm in their surroundings does them no good:
Their psychological tossing and upset cause an accompanying
disturbance in the body and infect it with their disorder.*

—PLUTARCH, "MORALS—PHYSICAL QUESTIONS"
(AITIA PHYSICA), CIRCA 100 AD, (PEARSON AND
SANDBACH TRANSLATION, 1965)

The idea of sea air as culprit was persistent. Jumping ahead
1,500 years we still find much the same explanation:

> *The sicknesse of the Sea, wherewith such are troubled as first
> begin to goe to Sea, is a matter very ordinary; and yet if the
> nature thereof were unknowne to men, we should take it for
> the pangs of death, seeing how it afflicts and torments while it
> doth last, by the casting of the stomacke, paine of the head,
> and other troublesome accidents. But in truth this sicknesse so
> common and ordinary happens unto men by the change of the
> ayre and Sea. For although it be true that the motion of the
> Ship helpes much . . . yet the proper and naturall cause, is the
> ayre and the vapours of the Sea, the which doth so weaken
> and trouble the body and the stomacke, which are not accus-
> tomed thereunto, that they are wonderfully moved and
> changed. . . .*

—JOSEPH ACOSTA, 1588, RECORDED IN SAMUEL
PURCHAS, *PURCHAS HIS PILGRIMES*, 1625

Even when motion re-emerged as a reasonable cause, scientists still didn't know precisely how it worked. Research focused
more on how to prevent or cure seasickness than on what caused
it. Today's scientists refer to hypotheses advanced in the 19th and
early 20th centuries as the *blood and guts* theories, since they usually involved either:

- changes in blood flow to the brain

- various innards sloshing around inside the abdomen.

In 1810 a Dr. Wollaston suggested the *cerebral anemia* theory
after he noticed that as a ship plunged up and down, so too did
the mercury in the barometers on board. Wollaston theorized
that the same thing happened to the blood in human arteries:

The up and down motions of the ship produced a periodic excess or shortage of blood in the brain, resulting in nausea.

This variation in blood supply was also a part of the *bouncing brain* theory, of which Dr. Carl Ludwig Schleich was a proponent:

> *The pneumogastric nerve may be irritated mechanically by rhythmic shocks of the brain, which is all too loosely hung in the skull. . . . The shaking of the brain may lead to a sudden convulsive cutting off of the blood supply, as indicated by Albert's experiment with hammer strokes on the skulls of animals. . . . Every up and down movement of the ship produces irritation after irritation in our nervous system, until the gradual accumulation of mechanical strains leads finally to a sort of "explosion." Seasickness is the final "reflex" of the vomiting center caused by rhythmic excitation.*
>
> —SCIENTIFIC AMERICAN, 1912

Try this. Shake your head from side to side. Now hit yourself in the head with a hammer. Dizzy? Want to throw up? Who needs more proof than that?

Another doctor (who suffered greatly at sea) had a theory that highly intelligent people were especially subject to seasickness. He thought that smarter people had softer brains, which were more sensitive to being tossed about in the skull. Those of us who suffer wholeheartedly endorse this theory. I'm sure *I* would score a perfect 800 on both the SAT (Seasickness Acuteness Test) and GRE (General Retching Examination).

In addition to the squishy thing inside your head there are lots of squishy things in your abdomen—guts—surrounded by various unsquishy things, like ribs and a diaphragm. As the boat moves up and down, these things move around inside you to varying degrees, jostling one another and jockeying for position.

> *As we rolled I felt that my internal economy was doing the same. At one moment all the moveable contents of the body, liquid and solid, were thrown one way, towards the feet, as it were; the next, they were thrown with violence upwards, and on the diaphragm, on the liver. This latter organ is so imprisoned under the ribs, so bound that it cannot get out of the*

> *way. Tickled, pounded, in this manner, it gets angry, excited,*
> *stimulated, pours out bile into the intestines and stomach,*
> *which ought never to receive it, except during the process of*
> *digestion, and this occasions sickness and vomiting.*
>
> —DR. J. HENRY BENNETT, *THE LANCET*, 1874

With your innards in disarray, you might end up with some empty space in your abdomen—the core of the *visceral vacuum* theory. As explained in *The Lancet* in 1887, the problem occurs if the vessel drops just when you exhale. Your diaphragm moves up to push the air out of your lungs, creating extra space. Your body drops faster than your innards, creating a momentary abdominal vacuum. Everyone knows how nature feels about vacuums: Vengeful nature makes you seasick.

To counteract the vacuum effect, Dr. Thurstan recommended holding your breath and contracting your abdominal muscles each time the ship dropped. Practicing this technique could give you a "strong" stomach, both literally and figuratively. In fact, seasickness has often simply been blamed on a "weak stomach."

> *On a certain ocean liner a great many of the passengers were*
> *sick. One young man in particular was very much worse than*
> *his shipmates. An elderly lady wished to be as sympathetic as*
> *possible, so walking up to the young man who was draped*
> *over the rail, she asked, "My dear boy, is your stomach weak?"*
>
> *"Weak stomach, nothing," he replied. "Ain't I getting as*
> *much distance as anyone?"*
>
> —OLD JOKE

With this in mind, lunch-tossing could become a formal part of cruise ship activities, with prizes awarded for distance and style. With health concerns curtailing tobacco-spitting contests and dwindling farmland constipating cow chip–tossing competitions, it could become the participatory sport of the 90s—maybe even an Olympic Event.

The internal billiards game your spleen plays with your liver and appendix was not the only focus. Researchers also looked at muscles strained by the ship's movement.

Dr. W. H. Hudson, traveling by ship, observed how easily seamen were moving all over the heaving decks while the passengers

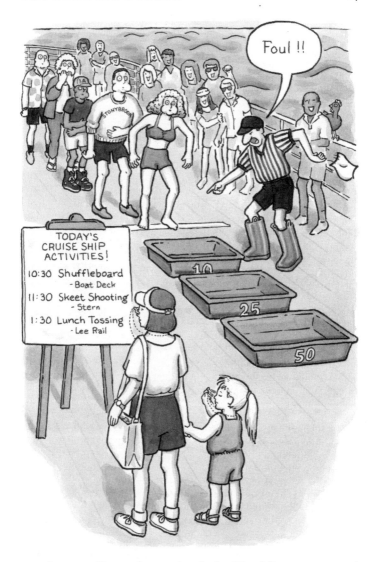

were heaving all over the moving decks. The difference appeared to be that experienced seamen didn't fight the ship's motions as did landlubbers. This profound insight led him in 1883 to write a book entitled *Seasickness*, designed to expose the source of the curse—muscular tension. The conclusions of his 136-page opus can be summarized in one word—*relax.*

Hudson was not alone in these ideas.

> *Sea-sickness is a direct result of muscular disappointments and nervous perplexities, arising from the unaccustomed efforts to regulate locomotion, respiration, and vision with respect to the novel and extremely unsettled state of things on the ship.*
> — STEVENS, *SCRIBNER'S MONTHLY*, 1883

Others blamed seasickness on more specific muscles, usually the ones that control the position of the eyes. Erasmus Darwin, grandfather of the seasick Charles, wrote in his work *Zoönomia* in 1794 that seasickness was due to visual disturbances. These theories failed to explain certain observations:

> *The notion that sea-sickness is entirely due to a disturbance of vision by continual changes of place in objects is shaken by the fact that blind persons are as subject to the affliction as those who see.*
> — ANONYMOUS, *THE LANCET*, 1843

This is not to say that vision is not involved in seasickness. Closing the eyes is recommended time and time again as a way of relieving symptoms, and it really does help.

A major breakthrough in finding the *real* culprit came from the work of William James, a psychologist at Harvard University in the late 1800s. While studying the deaf at the Perkins School for the Blind in Watertown, Massachusetts, he discovered that those with damaged vestibular systems, the balance organs in the inner ear, were not subject to motion sickness. No amount of spinning or rocking would make them sick.

James' work led to the development of *vestibular overstimulation* theories, which held that when there was too much motion, the signals from your balance sensors overloaded the brain. One big problem with these theories is that it is possible to have motion sickness without motion—what is known as *Cinerama sickness*. Watching a film shot from a moving platform such as a plane, a boat, or a roller coaster can make some viewers ill. In these cases motion sickness seems to be *entirely* due to vision.

All this is tied together by the *sensory conflict theory*, which

BRAIN

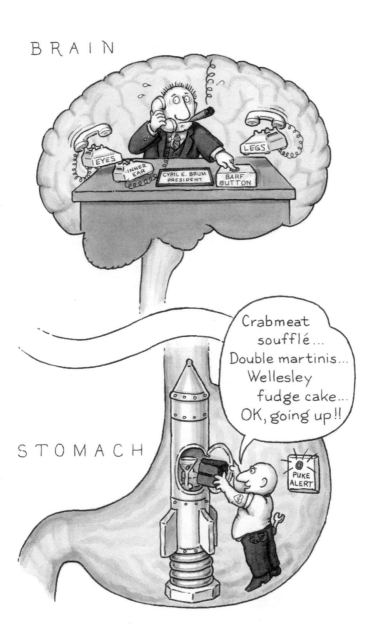

STOMACH

says that your brain receives information from various sense organs—primarily your eyes, your vestibular system, and the nerves that report what your muscles and joints are doing—about how your body is oriented and how it's moving. As we move about under our own power we develop a memory bank of normal combinations of signals.

Stimuli that do not fit the normal pattern produce conflict. If the conflict persists, the result is dizziness, nausea, and all the

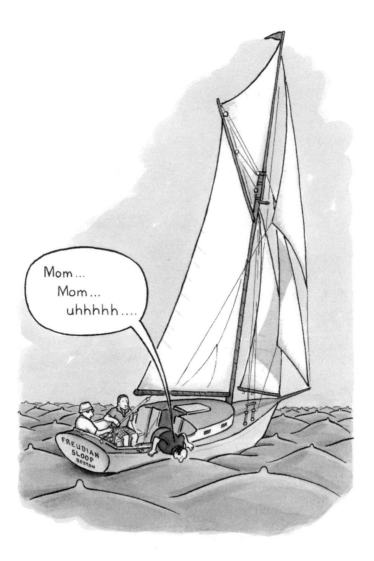

rest of that nasty stuff. While watching a film your inner ear tells
you that you aren't moving, but your eyes convey a different
message. When you go below on a boat the situation is reversed.
The objects around you don't appear to be changing their position, but your inner ear senses motion.

The conflict theory explains why most people, if they are seasick at all, are seasick only at the start of a trip. As you continue
to experience the motions, your brain's idea of what is normal
changes to suit the situation, and the conflict is resolved. You
have adapted to the new rules of motion and can enjoy the rest
of your voyage; you have your sea legs.

Perhaps the all-time best theory for the cause of seasickness allows you to place the blame on someone else—your *mother*. Leave
it to a psychoanalyst to come up with this one:

> Medical psychologists are familiar with dozens of ways in
> which patients associate the sea with their mother—in other
> words, the sea is a mother symbol. For our present purpose we
> need only refer to one of these associations—viz., the respira-
> tory rise and fall of the mother's breast while the child is tak-
> ing food. The rise and fall of a boat during a sea voyage tends
> to remind certain people of this forgotten situation in an un-
> conscious way, and sea-sickness with its rejection of food is a
> mode of repressing this infantile memory.
>   —W. H. B. STODDART, *THE LANCET*, 1924

CHAPTER 3

PICKLED ONIONS, ANYONE?
Remedies, Home and Otherwise

*The great bane of the ocean voyage is seasickness. The
infallible remedy for it is yet to be found. Its mysteries
defy the doctors and delight the cranks. Let your friends
know you are going abroad and you will be told of
enough medicines to stock a hospital. The most opposite
methods of diet will be advised, one man telling you to
eat all you can, the next advising temporary starvation.*
— ROBERT LUCE, *GOING ABROAD?*, 1897

These words still ring true 100 years later. Why are there so
many different, even contradictory "perfect" solutions to one
problem? Anyone who has ever tried anything that worked,
even once, is convinced that it is *the* remedy. Out of a sense of
humanity, or profit, they feel obligated to tell the rest of the
world. But did it work because it *did* something, or did it work
because they believed it would?

The truth is that absolutely *everything* can be an effective cure
for seasickness. No exceptions. All remedies can be divided into
two classes:

Physical cures

Remedies that work by some direct action on the body,
whether by suppressing nausea, affecting the sense organs
to reduce sensory conflict, or eliminating the motion entirely through mechanical devices.

Tinkerbell cures

Clap your hands, everyone. If you believe they work, they really do.

During an attack of sea-sickness one remedy is as good as another if taken with confidence.
— DR. BENNETT, *BRITISH MEDICAL JOURNAL*, 1928

Testing seasickness remedies

How can you tell whether a cure works for *you*? Let's say you try a remedy and you don't become seasick. So what? Maybe you wouldn't have been affected anyway on that particular boat with that particular day's weather. So was it the remedy? Or was it just getting a good night's sleep or having something different for breakfast?

These uncertainties create a problem for researchers. Tests on individuals aren't reliable, so they have to work with large numbers of people and rely on the VP (vomiting percentage) to identify effective remedies. As you can imagine, finding large numbers of willing subjects is not easy.

One doctor wanted to test the value of sodium nitrite as a cure for people who had already become seasick.

When Dr. Hayden was going to take a trip abroad he sought to put his theory to the test, but none of the passengers on the trip going over the Atlantic accommodated him by becoming ill. On the return voyage, however, he had better luck.
— *SCIENCE*, 1928

Seasickness has always been a hazard of seaborne military operations. Throughout World War II British researchers experimented with various drugs in order to reduce the effects of this problem on troop landings. With armies at their command, they had no problem finding "volunteers," but the weather didn't always cooperate.

Dependence on so fickle an element for experimental conditions imposed a considerable strain on the patience of the investigator. Chronic sufferers from seasickness may be astonished to learn that on most days throughout the year an obstinate and baffling calm haunts the waters around this island.
— HOLLING, MCARDLE AND TROTTER,
THE LANCET, 1944

The search for a cure

Everything that can be swallowed has been claimed to cure motion sickness.

— BRITISH MEDICAL JOURNAL, EDITORIAL, 1952

A list of all the medications that have been tested and promoted as seasick preventives or cures would read like the Merck Index. It would take less ink to list all the remedies that have *not* been tried at one time or another. In the interest of brevity, we'll limit ourselves to a select few.

- In 1837 Dr. Maddock said that a creosote [the stuff smeared on telephone poles] pill had worked well for him. He admitted that it had just one small drawback: The pill's taste was so awful that it made you sick.

- In 1857 Dr. Landerer recommended 10 to 12 drops of chloroform in water. Apparently if you're unconscious you won't care if you're seasick.

- In 1885 Dr. Wicherkiewicz prescribed a 5 percent solution of cocaine, to be started before the voyage. In the same year Dr. Manasseïn proposed a mixture of cocaine, wine, and distilled water, a teaspoonful every few hours for both adults and children.

And while we're flouting the Just-Say-No campaign, we should mention that opium has been recommended, both as a medicine taken internally:

If any palliative be given, it should be large doses of ammonia with opium.

— STEVENS, THE LANCET, 1838

or externally as an opium plaster on the pit of the stomach.

In simpler times one could buy a remedy that would cure not only seasickness, but anything else that ailed you.

Various herbal concoctions have been proposed as remedies. An ancient medical text prescribes:

DR. PETER'S

VEGETABLE ANTI-BILIOUS PILLS

When taken according to the directions accompanying them, they are highly beneficial in the prevention and cure of Bilious Fevers, Fever and Ague, Dyspepsia, Liver-complaints, Sick Headache, Sea Sickness, Jaundice, enlargement of the Spleen, Piles, Cholic, Female obstructions, and in all cases of torpor of the bowels, where a Cathartic or an Aperient is needed.

— ADVERTISEMENT, *CHARLESTON MERCURY*, 1838

So that you will not become sick on a ship:
Grind fleabane and wormwood together in olive oil and vinegar, and rub on the nostrils frequently.
— PSEUDO-APULEIUS PLATONICUS, *HERBARIUS*, 2ND
CENTURY AD

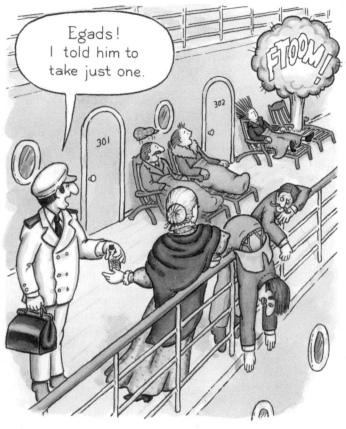

Nitroglycerin, so useful against heart attacks, has been used against seasickness.

A modern author suggests carrying a nutmeg in your trouser pocket, while from an older source we have a remedy accidentally discovered by a smuggler:

> *I remember a certaine Englishe-Man, who, when he went to sea, carried a Bagge of Saffron next to his Stomach, that he might conceale it, and so escape custome; And whereas he was wont to be always exceeding sea-sick; At that time he continued very well, and felt no provocation to vomit.*
> — SIR FRANCIS BACON, *HISTORIA VITAE ET MORTIS,*
> 1623

The discovery of Dramamine

Like many medical and scientific advances, the discovery of Dramamine's effectiveness against motion sickness was largely accidental. In Baltimore in 1947 Drs. Leslie N. Gay and Paul E. Carliner of the Allergy Clinic of Johns Hopkins University and Hospital were using dimenhydrinate, a synthetic antihistamine, to treat a pregnant woman with hives.

This particular woman also happened to suffer from an extreme sensitivity to motion sickness. One day she remarked to the doctors that she didn't become sick on the streetcar ride to the clinic after taking the new medication. The significance of this offhand observation was not lost on the physicians. They immediately contacted the army, and in November of that same year the drug received its first clinical test—Operation Seasickness—on board the troopship USAT *General Ballou*, bound from New York to Bremerhaven, Germany, with 1,376 passengers. The test was a success and led to the widespread use of dimenhydrinate to prevent motion sickness, under the trade name Dramamine.

The spice that has by far the best reputation is ginger, taken in any form.

- swallow ginger pills
- chew ginger root
- eat gingerbread
- drink ginger ale
- watch a Ginger Rogers movie

Some sources advise you to have a full stomach when you go to sea, while others advise you to fast. Since fasting is no fun, here are some enticing culinary recommendations for you to experiment with (more in Chapter 6).

> *Take a fish that has been found in the stomach of another fish, cook it, season with pepper, and eat it as you go on board.*
> — QUOTED BY DR. G. H. NIEWENGLOWSKI IN
> *SCIENTIFIC AMERICAN* SUPPLEMENT, 1909

- poke a finger into a bread roll, pour in Worcestershire or Tabasco, and eat quickly

- eat powdered charcoal after each meal

- a soup of horseradish and rice garnished with red herrings and sardines

- a small portion of beef, well chewed, as your only food, three times per day for the first three days out

- stewed tomatoes eaten cold with saltines

- a handful of salted peanuts at breakfast each morning

- sweet wholemeal malt biscuits spread with fresh butter, with a large chunk of mousetrap cheese, the whole well soused in Worcestershire sauce

- suck on fresh lemons

- essence of peppermint on lumps of sugar

Eating garlic on bread was popular among many European immigrants as a way of warding off seasickness. This diet reportedly did nothing to enhance the atmosphere in steerage, although it did reduce vampirism.

There is evidence to indicate that egg whites may do the trick.

> *Albumen is the only real cure that we have ever found in sea-sickness, for when nothing else will remain in the stomach, eggs, boiled as hard as possible, will! There can be nothing, perhaps, more indigestible in a healthy stomach than hard boiled eggs, yet in a sea-sick stomach there is no remedy we have ever found so potent. Eat from two to four and try them.*
> —JAMES ARLINGTON BENNET, M.D., LL.D., *THE ART
> OF SWIMMING, FROM WHICH BOTH SEXES MAY
> LEARN TO SWIM AND FLOAT ON THE WATER; AND*

RULES FOR ALL KINDS OF BATHING, IN THE
PRESERVATION OF HEALTH, AND CURE OF DISEASES:
WITH THE MANAGEMENT OF DIET FROM INFANCY TO
OLD AGE, AND A VALUABLE REMEDY AGAINST
SEA-SICKNESS, 1846

If eating and seasickness don't go together in your mind, you can always resort to drink.

A small teaspoonful of Cayenne pepper, diluted in warm liquid, sweetened, and taken as soon as the sensation of the complaint occurs.

— ANONYMOUS, *THE LANCET*, 1839

Take a handful of green wheat or grass, pound it, pour a little water on it, press out the juice, and let the patient drink a spoonful every 10 minutes.

— FROM AN UNDATED HANDWRITTEN MANUSCRIPT, MYSTIC SEAPORT MUSEUM

The sea will not cause nausea in anyone who has drunk a mixture of wine beforehand.

— MEDICAL MONKS OF SALERNO, *REGIMEN SANITAS SALERNITANUM*, 12TH CENTURY AD

Bicarbonate of soda in cold water, with three drops of peppermint.

— CAPT. VICTOR SEIDELHUBER, *NO MORE SEASICKNESS*, 1935

The yolks of two raw eggs with an equal bulk of good brandy well beaten together. A teaspoonful every ten minutes.

— PARTSCH, *SEASICKNESS: PRACTICAL PRECEPTS FOR OCEAN TRAVELERS*, 1890

In Shetland, a drink of water in which is placed a stone found in the stomach of a cod, will prevent seasickness.

— ENCYCLOPEDIA OF SUPERSTITIONS, FOLKLORE AND THE OCCULT SCIENCES, 1903

Recumbent position, eyes closed, and a pint of beer, ale, or porter taken in six or eight doses at ten-minute intervals

— PARTSCH, *SEASICKNESS: PRACTICAL PRECEPTS FOR OCEAN TRAVELERS*, 1890

Drink absinthe on sea voyages to prevent nausea.
— PLINY THE ELDER, CIRCA 60 AD

At the first symptom that the boat is going to roll drink some saline effervescing drink, or a pint of champagne. Do not drink any alcohol, except champagne.
— BASIL WOON, *THE FRANTIC ATLANTIC*, 1927

> *There once was a young man from Spain,*
> *Who washed down his meal with champagne,*
> *In a futile attempt*
> *To make him exempt*
> *From seeing the same food again.*

Sometimes remedies, like a nice dose of vinegar and salt, are discovered by fortunate accidents:

On a recent aquatic excursion I was, as usual, very sick. I tried brandy, soda-water, coffee, &c., without the slightest benefit. A lady on board was using brandy and salt for some purpose which I did not inquire about, but by mistake she put the salt (a teaspoonful) into a wineglass about half full of vinegar. This I mistook for my brandy, which was by its side, and swallowed. In a few minutes I was delighted to find the sickness much abated, and on taking a second dose was perfectly relieved.
— "A FRESHWATER SAILOR," *THE LANCET*, 1842

Since the concentration of wealth into the hands of a few is not original with the Republican Party, it's not surprising to find history sprinkled with potions that only the rich and queasy could afford:

Paracelsus (1493–1541) and his followers, and all the other alchemists, leave mysterious, complicated formulas based on salt, alcohol, and of course — drinkable gold.
— PEZZI, "LA CURA DEL MAL DI MARE ATTRAVERSO I TEMPI," *ANN. MED. NAVALE ROMA*, 1951

These drink-related remedies may be best when carried to the extreme (The W. C. Fields Cure):

> *Another and very successful remedy followed by a select num-*
> *ber of persons is to begin drinking as soon as the bar is opened*
> *and continue the treatment until you are in a condition when*
> *such sickness as ensues may be rightly attributed otherwise*
> *than to the motion of the ship. It is a curious but exact fact*
> *that very few confirmed topers are troubled by seasickness.*
> — BASIL WOON, *THE FRANTIC ATLANTIC*, 1927

Theories about the cause of a disease can lead to ideas about how to prevent it. Is seasickness due to your innards sloshing around? Well, stop them. How? Squeeze them together of course.

> *It is found by experience that if the abdominal muscles can be*
> *kept in an almost continuous state of contraction, the tendency*
> *to sea-sickness is very much lessened.*
> — DR. NUNN, *THE LANCET*, 1881

If only there wasn't so much elbow room for those innards. People have tried to solve this problem from both the inside and the outside. Bubbly drinks like champagne have often been advocated as a preventive measure, but the same Dr. Nunn suggested that:

> *The benefit resulting from these is due, I think, to the liber-*
> *ated carbonic acid gas; this gives pressure and support to the*
> *abdominal organs from within, and renders them less liable to*
> *be depressed.*
> — DR. NUNN, *THE LANCET*, 1881

In 1887 a Dr. Thurstan recommended eating pickled onions before a voyage, theorizing that the resulting gas would squeeze your innards together.

A more practical and reliable way of pressurizing your abdominal organs had been available since 1853, when Dr. Levilly invented the Thalaszone (from the Greek words for *sea* and *belt*) — a belt with padded steel plates front and back that could be tightened with a screw. The idea was that

> *being applied between the epigastric and umbilical regions, it*
> *maintained the viscera in such a state of immobility as to*

*prevent their friction against the diaphragm, and consequently
the retching.*

                    — LEVILLY, *THE LANCET,* 1853

The economy-minded might just don underwear several sizes
too small. Tight corsets have often been recommended, and

*some persons recommend a tight-fitting undergarment of strong
silk, but in order to be of use, it must be altogether too close
for comfort, and the wearer is quite likely to say that he con-
siders it the greater of the evils.*

                    — T. W. KNOX, *HOW TO TRAVEL,* 1887

The comfort issue was important even with the "scientific"
belts. A belt patented by C. Calliano in 1899 (US Patent 633,424)
was submitted to the medical journal *The Lancet* for testing.
They in turn gave it to a woman making a long voyage, who
wrote that:

*I buckled it on the first morning and found it most uncomfor-
table. I had to wear it without stays and I cannot say it was
anything but disfiguring and I felt qualms all day and after
dinner was very sick, so next day I did not wear the belt as I
thought I might as well be sick in comfort.*

In 1902, *The Lancet* editors added, in the politically correct id-
iom of the day:

*We fear that the disfigurement alluded to by our "tryer" will
be fatal to the extensive use of the belt by the female sex. If a
woman is sick in her cabin no one need see her, but if she is
seen in an unbecoming belt and is not sick she will probably
be more uncomfortable than if she were ill and unseen. But for
the mere man we think it very likely that in certain cases Dr.
Calliano's belt will prove very useful.*

While no marine supply stores or cruise-ship boutiques sell
anti-seasickness belts today, it's an idea that's been slow to die
out. As recently as 1984 there is a patent for a new version.
Over the years there have been a number of embellishments

to the basic binder belt. One doctor's version had multiple air sacs that the wearer could inflate with a built-in hand pump to produce the desired pressure. It had added benefits, too:

When the air-cells are strongly inflated, the belt is capable of sustaining a person in the water.
— NUNN, *THE LANCET*, 1881

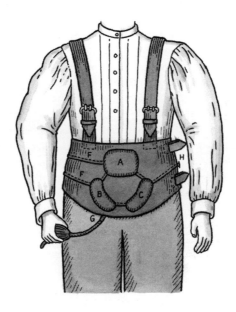

Another doctor suggested that in addition to the pads,

if a mild galvanic current could be passed between the two, a beneficial result would be expected.
— HARRIS, *THE LANCET*, 1887

If the pressure didn't do the trick, maybe the electricity would. Electricity has been used in other ways. In the 1930s a French researcher advocated using an electric neck heater to warm the medulla oblongata, the portion of the brain that was thought to be most involved in vomiting.

In 1985 a patent was issued for an electrical circuit designed to treat seasickness by stimulating the vestibular system with a series of pulses.

> *In essence, the invention provides this relief by producing in the afflicted person a sense of gravity acting on his limbs, thereby providing a perception of "heaviness."*
> — HERMANN MARK, US PATENT #4,558,703

The inventor suggests that the electrodes could be worn in a pair of glasses or a headband, or could be "implanted in or glued to the patient's skull area."

For those who favor the "cerebral anemia" theory over the "visceral vacuum" theory, here's a simple and inexpensive method:

> *Patient to lie down flat on the back, and fold a towel soaked in water, as hot as can be endured and as tightly as possible around the head, reheating the towel at intervals. This restores the proper circulation of the blood, relieves the abdomen from pressure, and checks the cerebral anemia.*
> — E. WOLF, LETTER TO *SCIENTIFIC AMERICAN*, 1907

A modern cure combats seasickness with the ancient technique of acupressure. Elastic bands with plastic knobs are worn on each wrist, applying pressure to the "nei kuan" points (three fingerbreadths above the wrist joint and between the two prominent flexor tendons going to the fingers) that communicate with the body's vomiting center. Like most seasick cures, they seem to work for some people.

In the mid-1800s Dr. Chapman of London developed his own theory to explain seasickness (and every other disease known to man).

> *I hold that the proximate cause of sea-sickness consists in an undue amount of blood in the nervous centres along the back, and especially in those segments of the spinal cord related to the stomach and the muscles concerned in vomiting. . . . The only scientific and really effective remedy for sea-sickness must be one which has the power of lessening the amount of blood*

in the whole nervous centres along the back. This can be
effectually done by lowering the temperature of the spinal
region by the application of ice.

—CHAPMAN, *SEA-SICKNESS AND HOW TO*
PREVENT IT, 1868

Chapman invented and patented the Spinal Ice Bag (US Patent 46,535, 1865), which required "from two to three pounds of ice for every two hours the passage lasts." As this was before the general use of refrigeration, especially aboard ship, it was not without its problems.

The early versions of his invention had other problems as well. One of the first to test the device wrote Dr. Chapman that:

> *the india-rubber in the lowest division gave way, and only a*
> *quarter of an hour after we started a hole was made, which*
> *allowed the melted ice to pour down my back. You can imag-*
> *ine what a pleasant feeling this perpetual stream was during a*
> *cold night.*

Chapman tried hard to have his idea accepted, and became frustrated that ships' doctors would not recommend his treatment, and that the steamship companies would not immediately stock their ships with ice. This led Dr. Chapman to form a new theory about seasickness.

> *It has been stated, on the best authority, that proprietors of*
> *passenger steamers are not likely to look with favour on any*
> *proposal to prevent the passengers from being sick, for that in*
> *estimating the cost of carrying them—across the Atlantic, for*
> *example—the fact that a certain proportion of them will be*
> *sick, and therefore without appetite for an average number of*
> *days during each passage is taken into account, and that were*
> *sea-sickness prevented or materially lessened, while the scale of*
> *fares remains the same, the profits of the proprietors would be*
> *reduced.*

If Dr. Chapman felt that a spine-chilling experience was an effective prophylaxis, maybe a brush with death would be even more effective—just the thing to pull you out of your misery.

In 1868 George Pierce sailed from Boston on the *Enrique*, bound for Australia with his wife, Elizabeth, and daughter Belle. George felt fine, but the ladies were continuously sick right from the start. When they were three weeks out:

> *About 2 PM as one of the sailors were slushing the mizzen mast 60 or 70 feet high he accidentally dropped the slush pot, nearly full of grease, weighing 6 or 8 lbs. and hit Elizabeth square on her left thigh, inflicting a severe bruise which is very painful but I trust not very serious. . . . Elizabeth had been quite seasick up to the time of the accident but the fright attending that seems to have entirely cured her.*
> —G. G. PIERCE, MANUSCRIPT JOURNAL, 1868,
> MYSTIC SEAPORT MUSEUM

The cure lasted for about a week. The critical element seems to have been fear. As we'll see in the next chapter, the mind and associated emotions play a major role in the question, to hurl or not to hurl.

> *. . . a storm at sea produced widespread sea-sickness, but at the first suspicion of real danger many victims lost all the despondency of sea-sickness in an ecstasy of hymn-singing.*
> —HILL, *BRITISH MEDICAL JOURNAL*, 1936

In times gone by, instilling fear in seasick sufferers was a routine treatment:

> *Long ago green midshipmen in the English navy had a rope's-end applied to them to stir them up to their duties, and sea-sick men on board whaling vessels had buckets of salt water dashed over them.*
> —CHARTERIS, *THE LANCET*, 1894

Many people, doctors included, believed that people with one eye were immune to seasickness; ergo, extreme sufferers of a nautical persuasion should have an eye removed—the Cyclops Cure. A bit radical, you say? Perhaps a simple eye patch would do

The plastic cure: a true story

Not long ago, during the annual Around Long Island Race, one member of a particular boat's crew became horribly seasick, but since the boat was racing, his fellow sailors refused to do anything about it. The sufferer resorted to waving his credit cards at passing vessels, attempting to purchase alternative transportation to shore.

The crew of one boat that came within earshot rebuffed him, saying, "Sorry, we don't take American Express."

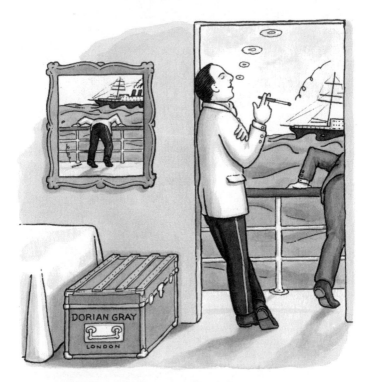

The Picture of Dorian Gray Cure

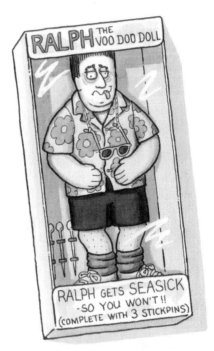

The Voodoo Cure

the trick. A correspondent to *The Lancet* recommended this as an infallible cure, with the added advice:

> *To be absolutely sure stuff cotton-wool into the opposite ear. . . . On D-Day, instead of fiddling about with hyoscine injections, the invaders could have jumped on the beaches tearing off red eye shades with one hand and pulling out blue ear plugs with the other. Perhaps the Germans would have thought this was the secret weapon at last and would have capitulated without resistance.*

> —ANONYMOUS, 1947

Unfortunately the "monocular cure" is just a myth. Admiral Nelson lost an eye in a battle at Calvi, Corsica, in 1794, but that didn't cure his seasickness. And a doctor who lost an eye in World War II wrote that:

*Anyone who noticed my pitiable state when the Channel
steamer reached Folkestone one day last October could only
conclude that I may have become a worse sailor but hardly a
better one.*
                          —DR. WATSON, *THE LANCET*, 1948

Maybe you'd rather sacrifice your hearing than your sight.
The inner ear plays a central role in sensory conflict, thus:

*In diseases of the internal ear a relative immunity to acciden-
tal disturbances might be expected, and, indeed, persons with
perforated drums, previously martyrs to sea-sickness, have
been freed by their disability.*
                  —BENNETT, *BRITISH MEDICAL JOURNAL*, 1928

Permanent damage may not be necessary. In a 1916 article in
The New York Times, Van Buren Thorne, M.D., described another doctor's experiment:

*He went out to sea purposely to make himself seasick, and
when in that condition he had a colleague of his douche cold
water in both of his ears simultaneously. . . This produced a
decided lessening of his seasickness. Unfortunately, for therapeutic purposes, the relief lasted only so long as the douching
was kept up.*

The simpler alternative is to stuff your ears with cotton. President Calvin Coolidge is supposed to have

*mixed a smidgen of science with his psychology; he plugged his
ears with pledgets soaked in tutocaine.*
                                          —*FORTUNE*, 1947

Treatments related to posture or manipulation of the body

*One of the circus performers who arrived yesterday from Ger-
many . . . was Goo-gu, the human pendulum, from the region
of the Yangtze, who entertained the passengers during the*

*stormy weather with his novel remedy for seasickness. When
the ship was rolling her gunwales under the chops of the
Channel, Goo-gu staggered out on to the upper deck and
suspended himself by his toes to one of the iron battens
athwartships, where he swung rhythmically to and fro for
fifteen minutes. Then he felt so much better that he was able
to eat pea soup, fat bacon and greens for lunch.*
— *THE NEW YORK TIMES*, MARCH 20, 1922

*Always go on deck when you are able to do so, even if you are
carried up by your friends or the stewards and deposited in
your chair like an armful of wet clothing.*
— KNOX, *HOW TO TRAVEL*, 1887

For short passages, one doctor recommended that you face in
the direction the boat is going, stand in a place out of the
weather but where you can breathe fresh air, and as the boat
rises on a wave, move quickly uphill.

*In this manner I deceived my stomach. That organ imagined
the motion was due to my own exertions, which it did not
object to submit to, and never found out that at the same time
that I walked or ran uphill the boat was playing all sorts of
tricks on me.*
— SUTHERLAND, *THE LANCET*, 1887

Here are some other published recommendations, which we
suggest you try all at once:

- lie down on your right side
- lie down on your left side
- lie down with your head facing the bow
- lie down with your head facing the center of the vessel
- turn your back to the sea when sitting on deck

According to many writers, seasickness can be combatted
through simple breathing regimens, but which to use? One
writer advises you to inhale when the ship rises and exhale when

it falls; another says to exhale when the ship rises and inhale when it falls. Take your choice. While you're trying to synchronize your breathing with the ship's motions, ponder this advice:

> Many a threatened sickness may be averted by a few deep, full inspirations at regular and rather rapid intervals. Under all circumstances the breathing should be strictly dissociated from the motions of the ship.
>
> —STEVENS, *SCRIBNER'S MONTHLY*, 1883

But why breathe just plain old sea air, which may be the problem in the first place? Far better to breathe something you can pay for. One such treatment was offered in the early 1930s by North German Lloyd on several of its ocean liners.

> The ship's surgeon, Dr. Dammert, offered the Dammert Inhalation Treatment for seasickness, price two marks. The patient had to inhale a mixture of oxygen and atropine, the oxygen to revive the system and the atropine to calm the nervous inner ear. This treatment could not, however, be administered in the cabin: it was first necessary for the sufferer to have the will to go on deck to receive it.
>
> —COLEMAN, *THE LINERS*, 1977

In 1941, an enterprising American doctor, Walter Meredith Boothby of the Mayo Clinic, invented a mask (US Patent #2,241,535) that allowed the wearer to breathe oxygen through the nose while leaving the mouth free for talking, eating, or smoking—although the latter might lead to a somewhat more explosive and permanent cure.

Of course, if one doctor suggested oxygen, another had to recommend carbon dioxide. According to a *New York Times* article from 1935, a Dr. Kerr blamed seasickness on hyperventilation, which could be stopped by breathing CO_2. If you don't happen to have a supply on hand, you can stick your head in a paper bag and breathe, or simply hold your breath for 15 seconds.

Invention has more than one mother, with necessity barely edging misery in the race to the maternity ward. Devices designed to diminish a ship's debilitating displacements have ranged from hammocks and cabins that isolate a traveler from the sickening motion to an entire seasick-free ship.

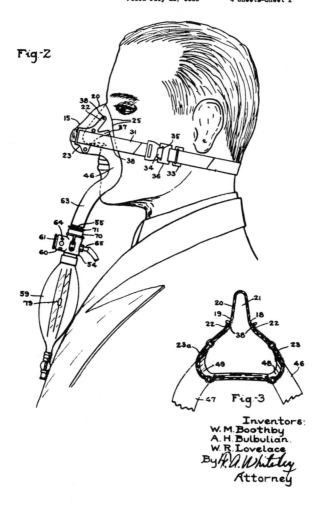

May 13, 1941.   W. M. BOOTHBY ET AL   2,241,535
APPARATUS FOR DELIVERING AND PERMITTING NORMAL
BREATHING OF MIXTURES OF GASES
Filed July 28, 1939   4 Sheets-Sheet 2

Fig-2

Fig-3

Inventors:
W. M. Boothby
A. H. Bulbulian.
W. R. Lovelace
By R. A. Whiteley
Attorney

The early 1880s were a busy time for companies like the Huston Improved Ship's Berth Co. and Miller Berth and Life Saving Mattress Co.—both of which produced berths that promised passengers a roll-free rest. No fewer than 29 U.S. patents for "self-leveling berths" were issued between 1881 and 1883.

For those who might not want to make an entire trip lying

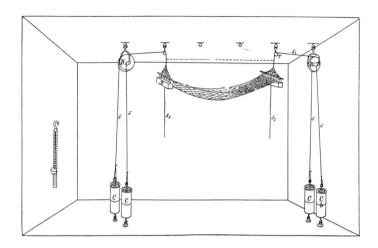

down, a patent was issued to Carl Brendel of Tschupackowka, Russia, for an oscillating chair.

> *In consequence of the long movements of the ship being thus changed into a great number of short motions which are constantly interrupted by short movements in an opposite direction the causes producing seasickness are counteracted.*
> — BRENDEL, US PATENT 769,466, 1904

Stepping up in size, *Scientific American* of 1912 refers to

> *construction of modern cabins on the more luxurious and expensive ships by means of swinging tanks, which causes Dr. Schleich to predict that eventually seasickness will be unknown to the wealthy, though "the greater majority of poor devils will still have to depend on their best friend, the ship's surgeon."*

After England's Sir Henry Bessemer earned his title, fame, and fortune as the inventor of the Bessemer process, an improved method for steelmaking, he was free to turn his attention to the much more important work of fighting seasickness, for which he had a strong personal motivation:

> *Few persons have suffered more severely than I have from seasickness, and on a return voyage from Calais to Dover in*

No. 769,466.   PATENTED SEPT. 6, 1904.

O. BRENDEL.

APPARATUS FOR THE PREVENTION OF SEASICKNESS.

APPLICATION FILED APR. 6, 1903.

NO MODEL.

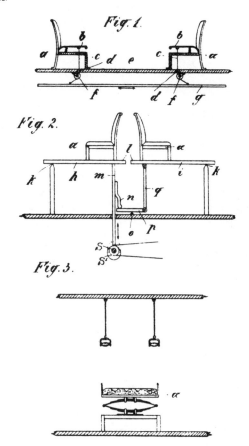

Fig. 1.

Fig. 2.

Fig. 3.

WITNESSES

C. P. Goepel.

John J. Little

INVENTOR

Carl Brendel

BY Goepel Vilas

ATTORNEYS.

the year 1868, the illness commencing at sea continued with great severity during my journey by rail to London, and for twelve hours after my arrival there.

— SIR HENRY BESSEMER, AUTOBIOGRAPHY, 1905

By 1869 Bessemer had a patent for a cabin mounted on pivots that would isolate it from the roll of the ship. By the time it was built the design had evolved into an elaborate salon 50 feet long, 30 feet wide, and 20 feet high, with a promenade deck on top.

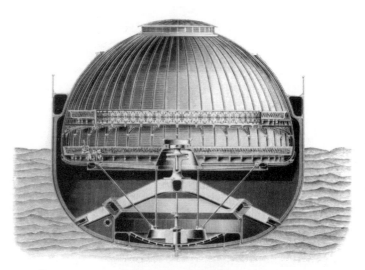

Fig. 81. Section through Early Form of Bessemer Saloon, in Still Water

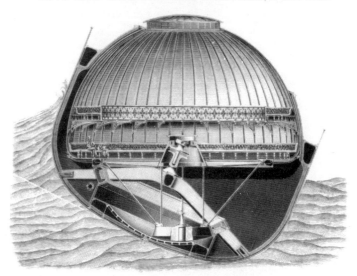

Fig. 82. Section through Early Form of Bessemer Saloon, with Vessel Rolling

Bessemer formed a steamship company and built a 350-foot-long ship specially constructed to carry the cabin. Hydraulic cylinders controlling the cabin's position would be operated by a crewman watching a leveling device. Bessemer sacrificed his health and a great deal of money in his efforts to complete the project. In 1875 the ship was finally ready for sea trials.

Unfortunately, the ship had maneuvering problems unrelated to the salon. On arriving in Calais harbor after its first Channel crossing the ship rammed the pier and was damaged. Returned to Dover and hurriedly repaired, the ship hit the pier again on the next crossing—this time with many VIPs and members of the press on board. The company went bankrupt. While some accounts say that the cabin rolled more than the ship did, Bessemer claims that the cabin was never tested in its proper mode of operation.

While few ships in the years since Bessemer have been designed from the keel up with seasickness prevention as the primary goal, a number of inventions that reduce rolling motions—moveable ballast, stabilizing fins, gyroscopes, and more—have been successful in calming this queasy mood. Today's passenger vessels provide a very quiet ride indeed.

But technology marches on. In 1991, a hotel chain built a cruise ship specifically designed to eliminate the threat of seasickness. The 410-foot-long vessel has twin hulls for increased stability—in other words, a catamaran, a hull form recommended by no less an authority than the U.S. Navy. In *Seakeeping Criteria and Specifications* (Naval Ship Research and Development Center, 1973), authors Hadler and Sarchin write: "A primary intent of this configuration is to attain high speeds in a seaway with small attendant motions."

Miscellaneous remedies

- traditional remedy for Scotsmen—a sixpence between the teeth
- clean the wax from your ears
- wear sunglasses
- put a Band-Aid over your belly button

- put mentholatum in your belly button

- expose yourself to ultraviolet light

- wear a piece of brown paper against your chest

- drink a good dose of sea-water

- lie in a tub of cold salt water

- lie in a tub of warm salt water

- listen to a Walkman (Debussy's *La Mer*, or the Red Hot Chili Peppers, depending on persuasion)

- no caffeine for two weeks prior to going to sea

- place bits of cracked ice in your mouth

- a hot water bottle over the stomach

- in the tropics, a lump of ice held against the pit of the stomach

- a calomel purge followed by a thorough saline irrigation of the bowels

- a few drops of camphor in water

- hot bottles to the feet and a shade over the eyes

- mustard leaves over the stomach and on the back of the neck.

In Iceland, a turf from a graveyard is thought to be a sure preventive of seasickness.
—*ENCYCLOPEDIA OF SUPERSTITIONS, FOLKLORE AND THE OCCULT SCIENCES*, 1903

Henry Sidgwick, English philosopher, . . . would choose a secluded corner of the deck and there declaim poetry at the rolling seas in a loud and expressive tone and with emphatic gesticulation. Given the opportunity, he could keep it up for a couple of hours. But the ship's officers would request him to desist. His behavior frightened other passengers into thinking him deranged.
—*THE NEW YORK TIMES*, 1936

As the head controls mental operations, a good massage at the
base of the skull close to the center of the brain nerves, is very
effective. Another practice—take a sharp comb and comb the
scalp for about ten minutes upon rising in the morning. Mas-
saging, as well as the combing, should be performed, if possi-
ble, by another person.

— CAPT. VICTOR SEIDELHUBER, *NO MORE*
SEASICKNESS, 1935

Celebrity endorsements

Whether diet plan, denture adhesive, or thigh shaper, few
things are marketed without the obligatory Endorsement of A
Luminary. Why should seasickness be any different?

George Bernard Shaw has a method of his own for preventing
seasickness, according to a letter in The British Medical
Journal. *By relaxing his muscles and allowing his knees to*
sag, he slithers up and down the deck of a rolling ship past
rows of green-faced passengers huddled in their deck chairs,
and never, so he says, feels the slightest nausea. The only
trouble with his remedy seems to be that it makes the other
passengers feel worse just to look at him.

— *THE NEW YORK TIMES*, 1936

Poet of the Sea John Masefield had this advice:

I think one of the best remedies is to drink a little salt water,
and frequently a piece of salt pork on a string will effect a
cure.

— *THE NEW YORK TIMES*, 1936

Lord Byron, apparently well-versed in the subject, wrote of
one way to settle a stomach in his epic poem, "Don Juan," circa
1820:

The best of remedies is a beef-steak
Against sea-sickness: try it sir, before
You sneer, and I assure you this is true,
For I have found it answer—so may you.

If you're cynical about the conflicting messages of celebrity endorsements, you're in good company.

> *Nor could they have avoided seasickness by drinking salt water (pure or mixed with wine) some days previously; or by using quince, lemonpeel, the juice of sourish pomegranates; or by fasting a long time and covering their bellies with paper; or by following other remedies that foolish physicians prescribe for those who go to sea.*
> — RABELAIS, *GARGANTUA & PANTAGRUEL*, 1552
> (JACQUES LECLERCQ TRANSLATION, 1936)

Charles Dickens was desperately seasick when he crossed the North Atlantic on a steam packet in January of 1842. This didn't prevent him from wryly observing the attempts of a fellow passenger to relieve his misery:

> *I remember that he tried hot roast pig and bottled ale as a cure for sea-sickness; and that he took these remedies (usually in bed) day after day, with astonishing perseverance. I may add, for the information of the curious, that they decidedly failed.*
> — DICKENS, *AMERICAN NOTES*, 1842

Mark Twain had a firsthand opportunity to observe the effectiveness of a custom remedy:

> *Thursday, 3:30 P.M. Under way, passing the Battery. The large party, of four married couples, three bachelors, and a cheery, exhilarating doctor from the wilds of Pennsylvania, are evidently travelling together. All but the doctor grouped in camp-chairs on deck.*
> *Passing principal fort. The doctor is one of those people who has an infallible preventive of sea-sickness; is flitting from friend to friend administering it and saying, "Don't you be afraid; I know this medicine; absolutely infallible; prepared under my own supervision." Takes a dose himself, intrepidly.*
> *4:15 P.M. Two of those ladies have struck their colors, notwithstanding the "infallible." They have gone below. The other two begin to show distress.*

5 P.M. *Exit one husband and one bachelor. These still had their infallible in cargo when they started, but arrived at the companion-way without it.*

5:10. Lady No. 3, two bachelors, and one married man have gone below with their own opinion of the infallible.

5:20. Passing Quarantine Hulk. The infallible has done the business for all the party except the Scotchman's wife and the author of that formidable remedy.

Nearing the Light-Ship. Exit the Scotchman's wife, head drooped on stewardess's shoulder.

Entering the open sea. Exit doctor!

— *SOME RAMBLING NOTES OF AN IDLE
EXCURSION*, 1878

There are two cures that really do work, and both are available without a prescription. One involves not going to sea at all:

The only cure for seasickness is to sit on the shady side of an old brick church in the country.

— OLD SAYING

But, like fasting, this is no fun. The other method can be just as effective: *go to sea.* The human nervous system is adaptable; if it's exposed to a new set of signals long enough, it will decide that those are normal. Voila! The seasickness is gone.

Cure through adaptation does have two disadvantages: You have to expose yourself to the very condition you're trying to prevent, and may become seasick along the way; the other is the specificity of adaptation. Different types of ships have different types of motions, so that the adaptation you gain on one type may not help you on another. The captain of a destroyer may become seasick on a ferry boat.

This leads us to propose an entirely new and original invention in the war against seasickness, which uses the adaptation approach to cure you of seasickness *in the comfort of your own home.*

Introducing

THE QUEASY CHAIR
The Adapto-Recliner for the Frequent Cruiser

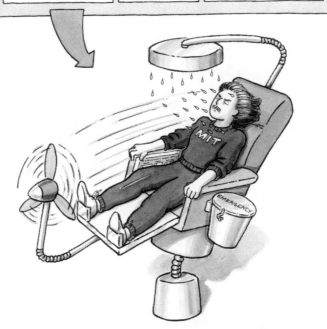

COMPUTERIZED CONTROL PANEL

VESSEL	MOTION	WIND VELOCITY
○ ROW BOAT	○ ROLL	○ GOLDEN POND
○ FERRY	○ PITCH	○ WINDBLOWN HAIR
◉ CRUISE SHIP	○ HEAVE	○ WHITE CAPS
○ PARTY FISHING BOAT	○ YAW	○ TEMPEST IN A TEAPOT
○ WHALE WATCH	○ CORKSCREW	○ HURRICANE
○ DESTROYER	◉ RANDOM	◉ POSEIDON ADVENTURE

The Adapto-Recliner Queasy Chair, designed by leading motion sickness researchers, allows you to build an immunity to seasickness in the comfort of your own home. One week before your scheduled voyage, just sit back and let the EasiAdjust onboard computer put you through a regimen of motions that replicate the motions of the boat you'll be on, and the weather conditions you expect to encounter. By the time you're ready to sail, you'll have your sea legs—all without leaving your home.

CHAPTER 4

MIND OVER STOMACH, STOMACH OVER MIND
Psychology and Seasickness

If you want to make seasick sufferers *really* mad—whether they're in the please-kill-me-now phase or just feeling a bit queasy—tell them it's all in their mind.

We sufferers know better. It's really all in our stomachs—and probably not for long. The rivalry between the susceptible and the immune is just one of the entertaining psychological aspects of seasickness.

> *The victim of the wretched malady was regarded with loathing by those of his fellow-passengers who were inclined to be sick themselves, and with contempt by the few who felt perfectly well.*
>
> —JAMES OWEN HANNAY, *SPILLIKINS*, 1926

While anyone can become seasick if the right conditions persist, it's human nature for those who are not seasick to feel superior to those who are.

> *By some happy fortune I was not seasick. That was a thing to be proud of. I had not always escaped before. If there is one*

thing in the world that will make a man peculiarly and insuf-
ferably self-conceited, it is to have his stomach behave itself,
the first day at sea, when nearly all his comrades are seasick.
— MARK TWAIN, *THE INNOCENTS ABROAD*, 1869

Seasickness is probably the only physical ailment to provide
pleasure to those who don't have it. It's like seeing someone slip
on a banana peel: It's funny if it isn't you.

I knew what was the matter with them. They were seasick.
And I was glad of it. We all like to see people seasick when
we are not, ourselves. Playing whist by the cabin lamps, when
it is storming outside, is pleasant; walking the quarter-deck in
the moonlight is pleasant; smoking in the breezy foretop is
pleasant, when one is not afraid to go up there; but these are
all feeble and commonplace compared with the joy of seeing
people suffering the miseries of seasickness.
— MARK TWAIN, *THE INNOCENTS ABROAD*, 1869

This enjoyment can turn malicious. Samuel Butler, the author of the utopian novel *Erewhon*, wrote in his *Note-Books*
(1874–1883):

I hunted the late Bishop of Carlisle with my camera, hoping
to shoot him when he was sea-sick crossing from Calais to
Dover.

You should think twice before gloating, for your own turn at
the rail may come when you least expect it.

One ov the best temporary cures for pride and affektashun
that i hav ever seen tried is sea sickness; a man who want tew
vomit never puts on airs.
— HENRY WHEELER SHAW (1818–1885),
ODS AND ENS

A young man, boastful and spry,
Felt queasy but would not say why.
'Til he swallowed his pride,
Lost it over the side,
Now he dines mainly on humble pie.

Just how bad is seasickness?

To put seasickness in its proper perspective, we must have something against which to measure it. What, for example, is any living creature's strongest instinct? Sex, you say? Come on, this is the 90s. The correct answer is survival—self-preservation. Millions of years of evolution have honed this instinct to a keen edge; it underlies everything we do. Nothing is stronger. Except seasickness.

The proof? In less than half an hour of seasickness, even a terminally perky alumnus of Up With People can mutate into a sniveling lump of green misery, praying for shipwreck or death. Fear of dying is transformed into an even stronger fear of living.

> *I had mal de mer once, aboard a private yacht. If somebody had killed me I would have made him my sole heir.*
>
> —MILTON BERLE

To measure the severity of an attack of *mal de mer*, ask the sufferer (or yourself, as the case may be) how bad it is. If the answer is that you're afraid of dying, stop worrying—it's just a mild case. But if you're afraid of living, the affliction is severe.

> *In some patients the mental effect is slight; in others there is a strong conviction that death is imminent, followed, as time goes on, by an unreasonable annoyance at its delay.*
>
> —BENNETT, *BRITISH MEDICAL JOURNAL*, 1928

> *As the ship and I tossed on a wave,*
> *And my stomach had naught left to save.*
> *I let out with a shout*
> *"Twould be better, no doubt,*
> *To be lying quite still in my grave."*

Lucius Annaeus Seneca (4 BC–65 AD) was a prominent Stoic, an advocate of the philosophy of enduring hardships without complaint, of accepting whatever hand fate might deal. In his *Moral Essays* he wrote:

Make up your mind that there are many things which you must bear. Is anyone surprised that he is cold in winter? That he is sick at sea? That he is jolted about on the road? The mind will meet bravely everything for which it has been prepared.

— SENECA, "DE IRA," (BASORE TRANSLATION, 1928)

But did Seneca live up to his own teachings?

I wonder whether there is anything I could not be talked into now after letting myself be persuaded recently into taking a trip by sea. It was calm when we cast off, and I thought it would be possible to make it across the few miles of water from Parthenope (Naples) to Puteoli (Pozzuoli), rather than following the winding coastal road. But when I had got so far across that it made no difference whether I went on or turned back the smoothness which had tempted me to my undoing disappeared. There was no storm as yet, but a heavy swell was running and the waves were getting steadily rougher.

I asked the helmsman to put me ashore somewhere. He said the coast was a rugged one, without a harbor anywhere. I was in far too bad a way, though, for any thought of danger to enter my head, as I was suffering the torments of that slow kind of seasickness that will not bring one relief—the kind that upsets the stomach without clearing it. So I put pressure on him and compelled him to make straight for the shore.

Once we were close in there was no more waiting on my part. I dived right into the sea in my clothes. You can imagine what I suffered as I crawled out over the rocks, struggling to safety. What I went through because of my inability to endure my seasickness is beyond belief.

You can take it from me that the reason Ulysses got himself shipwrecked everywhere was not so much because Neptune was against him from the day he was born, but because he was prone to seasickness like me. It will take me twenty years to reach my destination, too, if I ever again have to journey anywhere by sea.

— SENECA, "LETTER 53," TO LUCILIUS (ADAPTED FROM CAMPBELL TRANSLATION, 1969)

Some people, when faced with the clear choice between sea-sickness and death, have consciously chosen the latter.

> *Cicero, having taken refuge on board ship, preferred to return to Gaëa and submit to the envoy of Mark Antony commissioned to slay him than undergo the misery of sea-sickness.*
>
> — THE LANCET, 1891

> *How seasick was I?*
>   *I was so seasick it was only the hope of dying that kept me alive.*
>
> — OLD JOKE

Well, maybe you won't die this time, but you can expect to be transformed, at least for the duration.

> *How holy people look when they are sea-sick! There was a patient Parsee near me who seemed purified once and for ever from all taint of the flesh. Buddha was a low, worldly minded, music-hall comic singer in comparison. He sat like this for a long time, and he made a noise like cows coming home to be milked on an April evening.*
>
> — SAMUEL BUTLER, NOTE-BOOKS, 1874–1883

We could all use a little purification now and then.

> *This is one of the compensations of the sea-sick. The extraordinary humiliation which accompanies their sufferings is very good for their moral characters.*
>
> — JAMES OWEN HANNAY, SPILLIKINS, 1926

Seasickness has certainly been the motivation behind many prayers and promises.

> *Poor Panurge, hugging the poop deck in misery and affliction, invoked all the blessed saints, male and female, as well as Leda's twin offspring, and the egg that hatched them. He would, he swore, go to confession in an opportune time at the most convenient place.*
>
> — RABELAIS, GARGANTUA & PANTAGRUEL, 1552
>   (JACQUES LECLERCQ TRANSLATION, 1936)

If all else fails, you can always hope for a miracle.

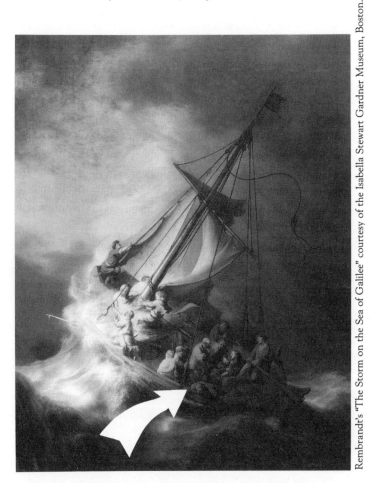

Rembrandt's "The Storm on the Sea of Galilee" courtesy of the Isabella Stewart Gardner Museum, Boston.

Apostle Ralph casting his bread upon the waters.

The truth about lying

Seasickness isn't always conducive to high moral standards. In fact, there seems to be a strong association between seasickness and lying.

*Me? I felt great! Everyone else was sick, though. I was the
only one who never missed a meal.*
                        — EVERYONE WHO HAS EVER BEEN TO SEA

Sound familiar? It's Denial. Ask any army veteran about
ocean crossings aboard troopships. Invariably, he was on board
with 10,000 other soldiers, sailing through the worst storms in
anyone's memory, and there was only one person on board who
wasn't sick. Guess who that was.

*It is a curious fact but nobody is ever seasick when on land.
At sea you come across plenty of people very bad indeed,
whole boat loads of them; but I never met a man yet, on land,
who had ever known it or what it was to be seasick. Where
the thousands upon thousands of bad sailors that swarm in
every ship hide themselves when they are on land is a mystery.*
        — JEROME K. JEROME, *THREE MEN IN A BOAT (TO SAY
                            NOTHING OF THE DOG)*, 1889

These people are carrying on an age-old tradition of sea travelers: Never admit you were seasick.

*If you should be so foolish as to be seasick, you must remember
never to admit it afterward. That is one inviolate rule never to
be broken. Unquestionably a good alibi is the only really
effective remedy for seasickness.*
                    — BASIL WOON, *THE FRANTIC ATLANTIC*, 1927

P.T. Barnum made the mistake of admitting it in print, in a
letter he wrote to the *New York Atlas* in 1844 after his first trip
across the Atlantic.

*I changed my wardrobe, and prepared for a long and dreary
time of sea-sickness, as I had fully made up my mind that I
should be sick during the whole voyage. This foreboding was
certainly but reasonable, inasmuch as I am frequently sick in
merely going up and down Long Island Sound.*

Barnum must have come to his senses after this egregious

breach of tradition: Just two years later, in a letter to the same newspaper, he denied *ever* having been seasick.

> *I have said nothing, thus far, of that class of passengers who are compelled every day to make a sacrifice to the fishes—to literally "cast their bread upon the waters." Happily, I have never been numbered among that unfortunate class, and am therefore incompetent to describe all their sufferings.*

A true practitioner of The Art of Denial would never be caught in such an error, and would not even admit it to himself.

> *A favorite amusement with them was to sit in the lee of the bulwarks, relating their experiences in former voyages—voyages distinguished in every instance by two remarkable features, the frequency of unprecedented hurricanes and the entire immunity of the narrator from seasickness. It was very interesting to see them sitting in a row telling these things, each man with a basin between his legs.*
>
> —AMBROSE BIERCE (1842–1914), *THE OCEAN WAVE*

And if you should ever get over your susceptibility, by all means deny that you ever suffered in the past. To help you carry on this fine tradition, we offer a number of ready-made excuses:

I'm not seasick . . .

I'm just hung over.

It's only a touch of the flu.

I think the chicken salad was bad.

I'm looking for a good spot to fish.

I'm looking for _____ (Jacques Cousteau, Lloyd Bridges, Jimmy Hoffa, giant squid, dolphins, sharks, Moby Dick, mermaids, the Loch Ness monster . . .).

I'm an oceanographer. I get paid to hang over the side.

I'm watching the submarine races.

Brain waves?

Seasickness clearly has an effect on the mind, but does the mind have an effect on seasickness?

> *I have often wished to see a convinced and skillful Christian Scientist in conflict with an attack of sea-sickness. There is no doubt that the disease is more susceptible than most others to treatment by suggestion.*
> — JAMES OWEN HANNAY, *SPILLIKINS*, 1926

Anyone previously cursed with seasickness is likely to be apprehensive any time he leaves the dock. Will I get seasick this time? Is that feeling in my stomach the start of seasickness? Or just the olive loaf? With seasickness, apprehension quickly brings on reality. Modern science even has a name for this: Anticipatory Nausea and Vomiting Syndrome (ANV).

> *Undoubtedly the chief predisposing cause of sea-sickness is anticipation.*
> — BENNETT, *BRITISH MEDICAL JOURNAL*, 1928

Claims of eliminating seasickness by mental attitude alone have been made. Dr. Benjamin Spock, the famous baby doctor and an experienced sailor, wrote of his wife:

> *On her first sail Mary got seasick. When I told her what it was, she said firmly, "I'm not going to be seasick anymore." And she wasn't. Mind over matter.*

Benjamin is not the only Spock involved in seasick cures. A correspondent to a boating newsletter wrote that, on a rough passage, he "overcame the heaves by emulating Mr. Spock. He imagined he was a Vulcan and seasickness was a state of mind."

A friend of mine, a laconic Southerner by the name of Walter Lee Eddins, once described an informal experiment he performed one rough day on board an icebreaker notorious for rolling. Many of the crew were suffering, but not Walter Lee, who positioned himself on deck near a hatchway leading to the rail. When an uncertain-looking crew member stumbled on deck,

Walter Lee adopted the guise of one who was about to run for the rail himself—invariably triggering the real reaction in his victim.

To vary the experiment, when one of the crew came on deck looking miserable, Walter Lee perked up and told him he looked great. The newcomer cheered up immediately, saying that he really didn't feel so bad after all. They conversed amiably for a few minutes, then Walter Lee changed his tack and told him that he was looking a mite peaked. The other fellow's expression changed instantly; in no time at all he was at the rail.

A good day of sport for the unflappable Walter Lee, Student Of Human Nature. Kids, try this one yourself on Mom and Dad.

The influence of the mind on seasickness has made it difficult to evaluate remedies scientifically. The placebo effect, where a person's condition improves even if he only *thinks* he has taken medication, can make any treatment seem effective. This explains why so many treatments have been promoted to combat the scourge of seasickness. Sure they work—if you believe they do (see Tinkerbell, Chapter 3). Not surprisingly, this effect has even been exploited for personal gain.

> *On a Channel steamer some years ago, a faker made a good living—until he was arrested—by selling bread pills to passengers, among whom was his wife, always the first who got marvelously well. Though these pills had no therapeutic value, it is a remarkable fact that many passengers actually felt quite well shortly after taking them.*
>
> *I have found with most people that seasickness is mostly imagination. If they are able to get it off their minds, and do not think of it, in most cases nothing happens.*
>
> —CAPT. VICTOR SEIDELHUBER, *NO MORE SEASICKNESS*, 1935

And so we find that it's easy to prevent seasickness: Just keep your mind on other things. Easier said than done. One common suggestion is to joke with (not at) the sufferer. Another is to give him some task to occupy his mind: coil ropes, count lifeboats—any straightforward job, preferably in the open air. *The New York Times* Sunday crossword puzzle is not recommended—nor is reading this book.

Strong emotions can also shift attention away from mere personal difficulties. Fear is nearly 100 percent effective.

> No one — at least no one who understands what is happening —
> is sick in a boat which misses stays with a reef of rocks under
> her lee.
>   — JAMES OWEN HANNAY, *SPILLIKINS*, 1926

Other strong emotions can have a similar effect. Anger works. Love has been recommended, but its power over seasickness has not been firmly established.

> How I should like to make love, if it was only for the fun of
> the thing just to keep one's hand in; but alas! all the young
> girls are sick — devilishly sick, and I trust I need not tell you
> that a love-sick girl is one thing, and a seasick girl another. I
> like to have my love returned, but not my dinner.
>   — THOMAS CHANDLER HALIBURTON,
>   *THE LETTER-BAG*
>   *OF THE GREAT WESTERN*, 1840

Of course there's always hypnosis. Your body may be at sea, but with a bit of watching the watch, your mind can be firmly planted on solid ground, leaning against that old oak tree next to the country church, with cows grazing in the rolling hills — no, better forget the rolling hills — with cows grazing on the flat plains stretching into the distance.

This is not a new idea. A 1901 note in *The New York Times* (the editorial staff of which seems inordinately interested in seasickness) says that:

> Seasickness will never be understood until it ceases to be
> classed as a physical infirmity and is rated where it belongs,
> among psychic phenomena. The best explanation of it which
> has come to our knowledge is that it is a disturbance of the
> nerve centres due to a lack of coincidence between the optical
> and physical sensations.
>   It is not inconceivable that the progress of science will
> ultimately find a method of bringing the optical and physical
> sensations into harmony. Hypnotism would seem to be the
> agency by which this can best be accomplished, and we won-

*der it has not suggested itself to the managers of the ocean
lines to supplement the services of the ship physician by those
of the hypnotist, who, by the proper line of suggestion, could
make those susceptible to seasickness fancy themselves free
from the conditions inviting it. Why should not those who find
a voyage dreadful from the moment the propeller begins to
revolve until the vessel is again tied to a dock, be made to
fancy that they are camping in the Adirondacks or abiding at
home in stable equilibrium.*

> Old Mesmer, the king of hypnosis,
> Was so sick his eyes would not focus.
> Swung his watch to and fro
> But that affected him so,
> That he retched from his head to his tosis.

In all of recorded history we have found only one case of anyone taking pride in seasickness. In early 1898, *The Sandusky Regis-
ter* attacked *The New York Times* for implying that intelligent
discussion of seasickness was "better left to the inhabitants of
States nearer the ocean than Indiana is." The writers of *The
Times* couldn't take this lying down.

> *If New Yorkers cannot lay claim to more knowledge on this
> subject than the Hoosiers possess, if they are not permitted to
> make so modest a boast as this, it is really too bad. And The
> Register is really severe with us, and asserts that nobody
> knows a tithe of the possibilities of the malady in question
> until he has sailed in the great lakes, especially Lake Michi-
> gan. We refuse to be shut up in this cruel way, and persist in
> believing that seasickness can be studied only at sea. Passen-
> gers on lake craft may endure frightful torments, but what has
> that to do with the matter. Lakesickness, we will admit, if
> The Register demands it, is much worse than any experience to
> be obtained on the Atlantic, but it isn't the Simon-Pure article
> at all.*

One would think that if "the Hoosiers" wanted to corner the
market on seasickness, they could have it. New Yorkers are not
so generous.

CHAPTER 5

~~~~~~~~~~

SEX AND THE SEASICK SAILOR
The Shortest Story Ever Told

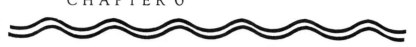

CHAPTER 6

SEA RATIONS
"You can't keep a good meal down"

An old African proverb says, "What the sea has swallowed it does not vomit out again." Unfortunately, this isn't always true for those who travel on the sea.

Food is an important part of the seasick experience. One way or another you'll be aware of it, whether you are:

- deprived of your favorite foods for fear you'll only possess them briefly.

- troubled by the food you just ate, which is waiting anxiously in the wings for an encore.

- disgusted by the guy at the next table with dried egg yolk (you hope) in his moustache and ketchup on his chin.

Just because you're going to be seasick is no reason not to eat. Although it sometimes seems an attractive option, dying of starvation is measurably more inconvenient than being seasick. But don't eat just anything. Your culinary experience can be greatly enhanced if you learn what dining at sea is all about.

And stay positive. The pessimist will say that seasickness means he won't enjoy his meals. The optimist will see it as a way to get twice as much pleasure from every bite.

Repeating repast is a natural phenomenon. At sea, meals simply obey a fundamental law of physics, first described hundreds of years ago by Sir Isaac Newton's seafaring third cousin, Ralph, who had a repeat encounter with an apple:

First Law of Nautical Gravity (Ralph's Law)
What goes down must come up

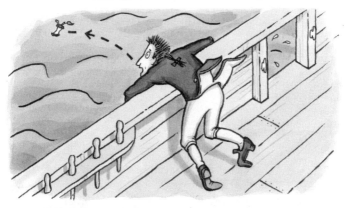

The unfortunate Ralph, feeling better and a bit hollow after losing his apple, attempted to fill the void with a full meal. A second trip to the ship's rail led him to formulate the Second Law of Nautical Gravity (Ralph's Law of Combinatorial Cuisine): It all comes up together.

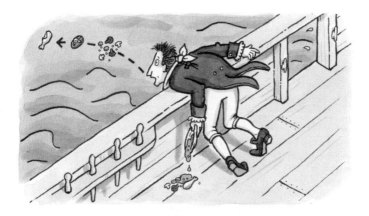

Suppose your first dinner aboard opened with *Potage aux Concombres*, followed by *Filet de Boeuf en Croûte* stuffed with *Foie Gras* and truffles, accompanied by fresh asparagus spears and a timbale of fresh corn. Wash it down with a good Bordeaux-Médoc, then top off the whole thing with baked Alaska and champagne.

When the S.S. *Rawhide* starts rollin' rollin' rollin', the individual courses won't all reappear neatly lined up in reverse order, like a video review of your meal running backward—no matter how well you chew your food.

Thus, the Second Law of Nautical Gravity introduces a new element into the art of ordering a meal at sea: planning for the future . . . *Your* future—staring into the briny deep with your meal once again on your mind, in your mouth, and before your eyes. Seasickness is a sensory assault, but with proper planning you can minimize the force of the attack.

Taste

> *There once was a man from Berlin,*
> *Who at sea always dined with chagrin.*
> *As he emptied his plate,*
> *He lamented his fate,*
> *"I fear I shall taste this again."*

Foods that are complementary as separate courses may be less so when combined on return. Would you mix together on the same plate:

- asparagus and peppermint ice cream?

- hot and sour soup and Roquefort dressing?

- oysters and cherry pie?

To avoid such unfortunate combinations, ask yourself *before* you start eating, "Could I stand this all mixed together in a stew?" Your answer should be an emphatic *yes*, because your stomach intends to do just that.

Why not save your stomach the trouble and make that stew right at the start? You can even experiment at home before your trip. Plan a meal, then throw everything in a big pot, mix thoroughly, and serve. The feedback you get from the rest of the family will quickly show you which combinations work and which do not. This technique has other benefits:

- it cuts down on the number of dishes to wash.

- it reduces time spent at the dinner table.

- it ensures good nutritional habits. Kids want to skip their vegetables and jump ahead to dessert? No problem.

> *A seasick old miser from Snee*
> *Took many a cruise out to sea.*
> *He was happy enough*
> *When the waves grew quite rough,*
> *For he had six meals daily not three.*

Vision

> *As in the case of drowning persons, there passed in review*
> *before my eyes several of the more recent events of my past*
> *life — meals mostly.*
> — IRVIN S. COBB, *EUROPE REVISED,* 1914

In addition to tasting your meal a second time, you'll also get to see it — and it's unlikely to have been improved by the experience. One way to minimize the visual impact, both for yourself and for others, is to eat dishes that look the same coming up as they did going down. This also saves you the trouble of playing "Name that Food."

Here are some foods that undergo little or no change in appearance after a round-trip on the alimentary canal:

scrambled eggs	macaroni and cheese
stew (any kind)	tomato soup
clam chowder	anything stir-fried
creamed corn	goulash
rice or noodle dishes	mashed potatoes

Strict attention to the proper techniques of seasickness (see Chapter 7, Seasickness as Performance Art) will help you avoid the added embarrassment of wearing your meal, but you should be prepared anyway. Eat foods that match your complexion (a somewhat sallower and greener version of it) or your clothes. Consider bringing along an assortment of food colorings to adjust your meal's tint as needed.

> *There once was a priest from Nairob',*
> *Who sailed off to circle the globe.*
> *On the first day he sinned,*
> *He faced into the wind,*
> *Now he's wearing his lunch on his robe.*

Feel

Would you eat a sandpaper sandwich? Then don't eat Grape Nuts if you expect it to repeat. Texture and consistency are much more apparent with food on its way up than on its way down.

Smooth foods are good, chunky foods are bad—especially *hard* chunky foods. You may experience every piece of fried rice, peas, corn on the cob, raisins, and alphabet soup at a time when you'd rather not, but at least they won't hurt. The same cannot be said for granola, popcorn, Cracker Jacks, peanut brittle, or double crunchy peanut butter.

At first glance spaghetti might look harmless, but picture yourself trying to *unslurp* a strand of spaghetti—through your nose. And let's not forget spicy foods. Even the briefest acquaintance with stomach acids will geometrically enhance the potency of chili peppers, hot salsa, or Szechuan cuisine. On their return your eruption will be truly volcanic.

Smell

For the other senses, careful selection of your food input can enhance the quality of your food output. This, unfortunately, is not true for the sense of smell: No matter what goes in, your nose will be offended when it comes out. All you can do is employ avoidance techniques—don't puke in enclosed spaces, and stay upwind of the seasick.

The food chain

When you dine aboard ship, you should take more into account than just your own petty needs. Although you may be hanging over the side, wallowing in self-pity and bile excretions, that's no excuse to be selfish. Who *really* benefits from your meal? Certainly not you. Think of others. Think of the fish.

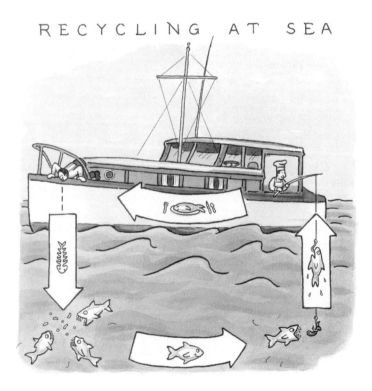

RECYCLING AT SEA

Panurge fed the fishes plentifully with the contents of his stomach, a fare these marine dungeaters absorbed with relish.
— RABELAIS, *GARGANTUA & PANTAGRUEL*, 1552
(JACQUES LECLERCQ TRANSLATION, 1936)

You may believe you're feeding yourself, but you're only a temporary way station between your plate and their stomachs — like a mother bird regurgitating partially digested food into the waiting mouths of her babes. Give some thought to *their* dietary needs. Don't fill them with mere empty calories, just because it tastes good to you.

> *At sea the food seems quite delicious,*
> *And I'm sure that it must be nutritious.*
> *I don't mean for me,*
> *It won't stay down, you see.*
> *I'm referring to feeding the fishes.*

The seasickness diet

If you still can't enjoy your twice-eaten meals at sea, look on the bright side. Didn't have the willpower to really cut back and lose those extra pounds? Now you have no choice. If you weigh the temporary inconvenience of seasickness against the continuous suffering imposed by the *diet du jour*, your outlook might improve.

In a 1912 travel article in *The New York Times*, Dr. Leonard Keene Hirschberg, AB, M.D. (Johns Hopkins) wrote that:

> . . . *for all its ludicrous horrors seasickness is by no means a dangerous affliction, and the great majority of ocean voyagers are benefited rather than harmed by the complete rest and total abstinence it enforces.*
>
> *People who are not seasick almost invariably eat too much at sea. The salt air makes their appetite prodigious, the hospitable steamship company gives them plenty of opportunity to nibble between meals, and the result is that they consume, on the average, twice or thrice their normal quantity of food.*

*The victim of mal-de-mer is protected from this impru-
dence. Instead of eating too much he abandons eating altogether. And for most normal human beings a few days' fast
now and then is a mighty good thing.*

Calorie counting at sea

Counting calories is straightforward on land, but at sea it's
more complicated. Food won't stay in your stomach long enough
to be fully digested, so you actually absorb fewer calories per
serving.

Food	Serving size	Calories on land	Calories at sea[1,2]
Hamburger	6 oz.	490	375
Bacon	4 slices	200	50
Fried chicken	6 oz.	300	100
Liver	6 oz.	280	27
Sardines	1 can	175	12
Saltines	8 crackers	100	100
Oysters	1 doz.	120	0.05
Diet soda	12 fl. oz.	just one!	−13.8

*1. These are average values. If you take your time getting seasick, you'll absorb
more calories. If you always tip the maitre d' to seat you at the table nearest
the rail, you may absorb fewer.*

*2. This includes an allowance for the energy required to propel the food from
your stomach and over the rail. This is not insignificant; you'll usually be
sweating as much as if you had just jogged through Central Park wearing a
wreath of hundred dollar bills.*

> *You may dine without guilt on board ships.*
> *Rich desserts may pass over your lips.*
> *Though you empty your plate,*
> *It won't add to your weight,*
> *And it won't spend a life on your hips.*

RALPH'S QUEASINE

"Food so good you won't care whether
it's coming or going."

UN-APPETIZERS

Stomach Turnovers
Delicate pastry shells
filled with your choice
of sea urchin roe,
baby eels, lumpfish
tripe, or anchovies.

Déjà Vu Fondue
Sooner or later, you'll
swear you've seen it
before.

Porthole Paté
Be sure you're near
one.

Presto Pesto
First it's gone . . . then
POOF! . . . it
reappears.

SOUP

Soupe de l'heure
Horseradish and rice soup,
seasoned with red herrings and sardines

RE-ENTREES

MacArthur Stew
"I shall return."

**MacArthur Stew
with Chili Peppers**
"I shall return with
a vengeance."

**See You Later
Alligator**
A Cajun-style favorite!
Deep-fried alligator
tail, garnished with
borrowed thyme.

Upchuck Roast

For the all-American
meat-and-potatoes
crowd.

Down Today, Up Tamales
The official food of popular uprisings.

Purina Trout Chow
For the unpretentious. You're just feeding the fish anyway.

All re-entrees served with

Tossed Salad
Eat a few lettuce leaves, a bite of tomato, cucumber, carrot, and celery. Wash down with a jigger of oil and vinegar. Wait ten minutes. Move to lee rail. Toss salad.

Rolls
and pitches and yaws and heaves

OVER THE SIDE ORDERS

Retried Beans   Splash Hash

JUST DESSERTS

Pineapple Upside-Down Cake
Served right-side up. Nature takes care of the rest.

Chocolate Mousse on the Loose
Careful, it might get away from you.

IN THE DRINKS

Pail Ale
Green Beer
Hakodate Highball
(as recommended by Mr. Moto in the film *Think Fast, Mr. Moto,* 1938)

All dishes can be ordered with FDA-approved food dyes in colors to match your attire.

SELECTIONS FROM RALPH'S SANDWICH BAR

The Play it Again, Sam'wich
It will bring back fond memories.

The Instant Replay Roast Beef on Rye
What the sports elite eat to repeat.

The Fundamentalist Foot Long Frank
Guaranteed to be reborn, with relish.

The Boomerang Burger
Just when you think it's gone for good, back it comes.

The Lazarus Sourdough Submarine
It always rises.

**The Honeymooners Ham and Cheese
(alias the Ralph Kramden)**
Great in re-runs.

The Orient Express
A chicken sandwich with Chinese-style sauce that comes up on you fast. You won't even have to wait an hour before you're hungry again.

The Yo-Yo Yogurt and Bean Sprout Pocket
The California curdler. Down, then up.

The Xerox Lox and Bagel
The duplicate is just as good as the original!

Mystic Pizza II — The Return
In the finest tradition of Hollywood sequels. Garnished with cheap sentimentos.

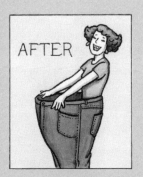

CHAPTER 7

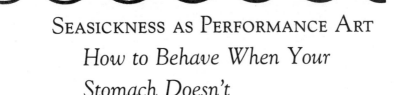

Seasickness as Performance Art
How to Behave When Your Stomach Doesn't

"My husband is peculiarly liable to seasickness,
Captain," remarked the concerned wife. "Could you tell
him what to do in case of an attack?"
  "That won't be necessary, Madam," replied the
Captain; "he'll do it."
                              —TOASTER'S HANDBOOK, 1916

So you're losing your lunch. That's no reason to lose anything else, like your glasses—or worse, your dignity. With just a bit of knowledge, common sense, and preparation you can exercise proper decorum before, during, and after seasickness.

First of all, prepare *not* to be seasick. You probably won't be. Follow the advice in Chapter 10, It's Not Easy Being Green. *Relax*. Assume you'll enjoy every moment of your trip, and you probably will.

But just in case . . .

> There was a young man from Ostend
> Who vowed he'd hold out till the end.
> But when halfway over
> From Calais to Dover
> He did what he didn't intend.
> 　　　　　　　—TOASTER'S HANDBOOK, 1916

Location, location, location

*If this is your first voyage and you are not quite certain about
the potential behavior of your stomach, a table near the door*

*leading to the first hatchway is indicated, and it may be wise
to practise between the table and the hatch a little before the
ship gets beyond Rum Row, just to see if you can improve your
time.*
— BASIL WOON, *THE FRANTIC ATLANTIC,* 1927

Wander around the vessel until you find a convenient and
easily reached site in which to be miserable. Ideally, it should
provide enough privacy to secure your own dignity, and to spare
your fellow-passengers a sight that might produce a sympathetic
reaction. Make sure it's a safe place, with plenty of rail to hold on
to; the combination of seasickness, seclusion, and rough weather
could have drastic results.

Rudyard Kipling used this combination in his book *Captains
Courageous,* the story of a spoiled rich boy who matures quickly
when forced to live and work aboard a Grand Banks fishing
schooner. How did a rich boy wind up on a poor fishing boat?
Seasickness, of course. Protagonist Harvey Cheyne, bound for
Europe on a plush liner, was showing off, smoking a cigar with
some of the other passengers. When the inevitable happened and
he needed to make a trip to the rail, his

*pride made him go aft to the second-saloon deck at the stern.
The deck was deserted, and he crawled to the extreme end of
it, near the flagpole. There he doubled up in limp agony, for
the Wheeling "stogie" joined with the surge and jar of the
screw to sieve out his soul. His head swelled; sparks of fire
danced before his eyes; his body seemed to lose weight, while
his heels wavered in the breeze. He was fainting from seasickness, and a roll of the ship tilted him over the rail.*
— 1896

Fortunately, Harvey was rescued by a nearby fishing dory.
Not everyone is so lucky.

The lee rail

Like Shangri-La or Fiddler's Green, the lee rail is something of
a mythical place—one you'll hear a lot about if you're feeling

queasy. The lee rail is defined as, *the place you must go—now—if you're going to be sick.*

But ships and boats have *lots* of rails—starboard rails, port rails, bow rails, and stern rails, but no permanently defined lee rails.

So where do you find a lee rail when you need one? The answer, my friend, is blowin' in the wind. There are certain activities one should never do into the wind; being seasick is very high up on the list. If there is no wind, then any rail is the lee rail. But the odds are, when you need to use the rail it *will* be windy, since wind makes waves, and waves make—well, we know what waves make us do.

So in your preliminary search for the lee rail, pretend (I know it's a stretch) that you feel great; you want to go out on deck, lean against the rail, and gaze out to sea, a fresh wind blowing in your face. Once you've identified *that* rail, you'll find the lee rail on the opposite side of the ship.

Conduct toward the seasick

As we pointed out in Chapter 4, Psychology and Seasickness, it seems fundamental to human nature to enjoy seeing *other* people suffer from seasickness. Fine. Go ahead and enjoy it. But play fair. Practices like these, though common, are considered unsporting:

- saying things like, "You think *this* is rough weather? Just wait until . . ."
- describing in excruciating detail the gourmet meals the sufferer has missed.
- eating smelly, greasy foods in front of them—and enjoying it.
- smoking anything upwind.
- making any references to Linda Blair or pea soup.
- taking their picture in a compromising position.

For your convenience, take along Mazel's Patented Lee Rail Locator

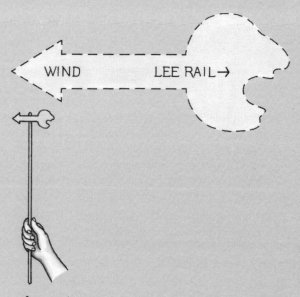

Instructions:

1. Trace the Lee Rail Locator onto a piece of cardboard and cut it out.

2. Color it green so you'll remember what it's for.

3. Mount the arrow on a thin stick so it's free to rotate.

4. Go out on deck and hold up the arrow. It will point into the wind.

5. Go the other way.

Warning for cruise ship passengers

You may not want to use the first lee rail you come to. Make sure that the one you find overlooks the ocean—not the ship's swimming pool the next level down.

- rocking back and *forth* back and *forth* back and *forth* back and *forth*

- bouncing

  up   up   up
    and   and   and   and   and   and over . . .
      down   down   down

And you should *never* play practical jokes on anyone, as in this *true* story:

> A Noted Marine Biologist and a World Famous Underwater
> Photographer were working together on a diving project in
> Jamaica. Between dives the Noted Marine Biologist was doz-
> ing on deck. The World Famous Underwater Photographer
> filled a bucket with seawater and left it to warm in the sun.
> When the water was near body temperature, the World Fa-
> mous Underwater Photographer made loud retching noises and
> poured the full bucket of water over the rapidly awakening
> and decidedly panicked Noted Marine Biologist. Many laughs
> were had by (almost) all.

If you're like most people, though, simple appeals to humanity and courtesy are wasted. But remember this: *No one* is absolutely immune; there may be a wave out there with your name on it. Your former victims might just do unto you as you did unto them.

Here's something else to consider: Abusing the seasick may carry more consequences than simply being swatted with The Golden Rule. William Bradford, a Pilgrim leader on the *May-flower*, wrote that:

> many were afflicted by seasickness. . . . A proud and very
> profane young man, one of the seamen, of a lusty, able body
> . . . would always be contemning the poor people in their
> sickness and cursing them daily with grievous execrations. . . .
> But it pleased God before they came half seas over to smite
> this young man with a grievous disease, of which he died in a
> desperate manner. . . . Thus his curses light on his own head,

*and it was an astonishment to all his fellows for they noted it
to be the just hand of God upon him.*
— BRADFORD, *HISTORY OF PLYMOUTH PLANTATION,*
1620–1647

So always have a kind and cheerful word for the sufferers.
Bring them some crackers or soup. Put a warm cloth to their
cold, sweaty brows. Try a little flattery: "My, that shade of green
goes nicely with your hat." It will do wonders.

The wearing of the green

Which brings us to fashion. Keep your sense of style. When
your inside is at its worst, your outside should be at its best.

If you follow proper seasick technique nothing will end up on
you, but you should be prepared for that missed step or sudden
wind shift. Select clothes that match your meal; alternatively, eat
only dishes that go well with your clothes and complexion.

If you've sworn off food entirely, you need only match your
complexion. The safest bet is a wardrobe entirely in shades of
green. Remember, at sea, every day is St. Patrick's day.

For those who insist on eating, come what may, one general-
purpose solution is to adopt a retro-60s look—paisley, or tie-dyed
tee shirts. These already look as though someone threw up on
them, so anything you contribute will go unnoticed, or may even
enhance the original appeal. You could, for instance, claim
you're wearing Jackson Pollock originals. This may not be a good
solution for everyone, however. A survey conducted by BLM
Opinions indicated that visual contact with some of these styles
will induce symptoms of seasickness in 17.6 percent of the popu-
lation while still on dry land.

Being sick

If something's worth doing, it's worth doing well. This is just
as important in being seasick as it is in writing the Great American Novel or cooking the perfect soufflé.

When the time comes, have some style. Excuse yourself with a
cheery wave and a polite phrase, such as:

Pardon me; I'm feeling the urge to purge. I'll be right back.

or

Would you mind holding my book? I'd hate to lose my place
while I'm losing my lunch.

Being sick need not even interrupt a conversation. Polite and
experienced sailors will deal with seasick members of the group
the same way people who live near airports deal with low-flying
747s. Everyone simply suspends the conversation, picking it up
again in mid-sentence after the event is over, as if nothing at all
had happened.

Know where the lee rail is. Remove your glasses in advance,
or tighten the safety strap. Remove your hat and false teeth.
Don't fight the ship's motion on your way to the rail. Allow the
roll to propel you effortlessly to, but not over, the side. The grace
and agility of your movements should remind onlookers more of
Mary Lou Retton and Olga Korbut than Joe Cocker or former
President Ford. This author once received two 9.7s, a 9.8, and a
10.0 for a roll-assisted transfer from the weather seat of a sailboat
to the lee rail, clipping on the safety harness en route and blowing lunch in a series of fluid motions.

It's one thing to be free of seasickness sitting in the cockpit or
up on the flybridge, with a ready view of the horizon and an end-
less supply of fresh air. It's quite another belowdecks in an enclosed cabin, with no proper visual reference to explain to your
brain the sensation of movement. Going below is *the* sure-fire
way to bring on a case of *mal de mer*.

Suppose you're out for a nice day of boating with a bunch of
friends. Typically, everyone on board is lounging contentedly on
deck, not a care in the world. No one is hungry. No one is
thirsty. No one needs to use the facilities. Hour after hour after
hour.

Innocently, you go below on some small errand. Bad mistake.
As soon as you start to emerge you'll be stopped in your tracks
by the most frightening words you can hear at sea: "While You're
Down There. . . ." Hot chocolate, tea, coffee, a sweater, a cap, a
candy bar, the sextant, make lunch — the requests will flow below
in an unending stream. You may not fully emerge until the boat

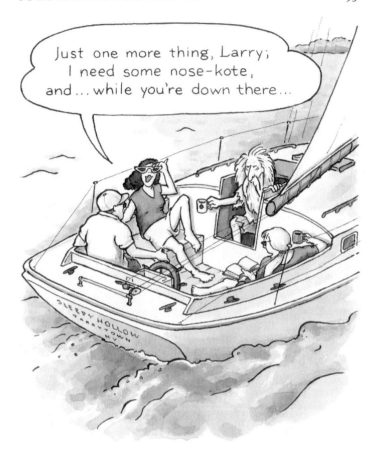

returns to the dock—unless you have to make a triple Axel for the lee rail.

Seasickness survival kit

The prepared passenger should have:

- glow-in-the-dark tape to mark the quickest path to the rail
- padded suction cups for your knees

- a safety belt that clips to the rail, with a foam pad for your stomach
- a bib
- scented nose clips
- cord for holding glasses
- hat strap
- a holder for false teeth
- wet-naps
- squirt bottle of water to rinse mouth
- packets of ketchup, mustard, mayo, and relish for camouflaging accidents
- blinders—so that you can enjoy the view without viewing others hanging over the rail
- skin-colored make-up—to cover the green
- Mazel's Lee Rail Locator to steer you in the right direction
- barf bag—in case you don't quite make it to the rail
- small squirt bottle of perfume—the cheaper the better
- Odor-Eaters

CHAPTER 8

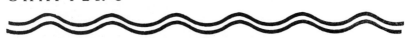

The Technicolor Yawn and Other Matters

Seasickness around the world

ALBANIAN - sëmunde prej detit (sëmunde—sick, detit—sea)

ARMENIAN - ծովահարություն
(tzov-a'-ha-rou-tyoun)

ARABIC - الدّوار البحر
(dawaran el bahr)

CATALAN - mareig

CHINESE - 晕船
(yun chuan—characters for 'dizzy' + 'boat')

CORNISH - cleves an mōr

CZECH - morská nemoc

DANISH - søsyge

DUTCH - zeeziekte

ESPERANTO - marmalsana

FAROESE - sjóverkur

FINNISH - meritauti

FRENCH - mal de mer, naupathié

GA (spoken in Ghana) - nshon hela

GAELIC - tinneas na mara

GERMAN - Seekrankheit (zay'-kronk-hite)

GREEK - ναυτια (nautia)
      με πειραζει η θαλασσα
      (meh pee-ra'-zee ee tha'-lassa) "the sea disturbs me"

HAWAIIAN - ka liliha ma ka holo moku ana (suffer sickness on a ship)
      poluea, luai moku (luai — vomiting, moku — ship)

HEBREW - מַחֲלַת יָם (makhalat yom)

HIEROGLYPHICS -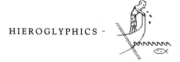

HINDI - समुद्र-अस्वस्थता (sah'-moo-dra a-vahs'-ta-tha')

HUNGARIAN - tengeribetegseg (ten'-ge-ri-bet'-eg'-shaig)

ICELANDIC - sjóveiki

IRISH - muirghalar

ITALIAN - mal di mare

JAPANESE - funayoi (fune — boat, yoi — drunk)

KHMER - pol ralok (poisoned from the waves)

KOREAN - 배멀미 (bae mal lai)

LAO - mao hya

LATIN - nausea

LATVIAN - jūras slimība (jüras — sea, slimïba — sick)

MALAY - mabok laut (mabok — intoxication, laut — sea)

MONGOLIAN - далайн долгионд толгой эргэн бөөлхс хурэх

NEANDERTHAL - buwaaaauggh

NORWEGIAN - sjøsyke

PALI (the canonical language of Buddhists) - sāmuddika-bhama

POLISH - choroba morska

PORTUGUESE - enjoado (nauseated)

RUSSIAN - морскáя болéзнь (mar-ska'-ya ba-lyeh'-zn')

SAMOAN - ma`ivasa

SANSKRIT - samudra rog

SPANISH - mareo

SWAHILI - ulevi wa bahari   (ulevi — dizziness, bahari — sea)
         kuchafuka tumbo chomboni — toss out your stomach
    contents on board a ship
    (kuchafuka — toss out, tumbo — stomach, chomboni
    — on board vessel)

SWEDISH - sjösjuka
         sjösjuk lätt bli — to be a bad sailor (become seasick
    easily)

TAGALOG - pagkalulà

THAI - **mao khluun**

TURKISH - **deniz tutmasi** (deh'-neez tut'-mah-seh)

VIETNAMESE - **say sóng**

WELSH - **clefyd y môr**

YIDDISH   yam-krankheit

ZULU - **isifo sokucanuzela esibangwa wukuhamba olwandle**

No matter what language you use, you should hope that it's only the *word* for seasickness that comes out of your mouth. Even if you stick to English there are any number of ways to say you're seasick. Noted sailor and litterateur William F. Buckley Jr., for example, would never say anything as plebeian as, "I got seasick and tossed my cookies." Instead, he might say, somewhat indifferently, "I suffered kinetosis and experienced emesis." Class.

For the rest of us, there are lots of popular options:

puke	hurl
spew	ralph
heave	woof
barf	upchuck
retch	toss your cookies
lose your lunch	spill your guts
feed the fish	blowing chunks
calling O'Rourke	driving the porcelain bus
making a sacrifice	
to Neptune	

We have the Australians and British to thank for these particularly graphic expressions:

technicolor yawn   liquid laugh   having a little spit

We can also thank them for *chunder,* the slang term for throwing up, derived from the words "Watch under!" This is what you're supposed to yell to people below, a lot like yelling "Fore!" when playing golf.

> Peter, a friend from down under,
> Says in his land the verb is "to chunder"
> When at the lee rail,
> If polite you will wail,
> "Heads up!", "Here it comes!", . . . "Watch under!"

Chunder can be used to describe vomiting in any situation, whether on land or sea. When aboard ship the strictly proper phrase is "chunder in the scuppers."

The terms "good sailor" and "bad sailor" have nothing to do with a person's ability to tie a bowline, box a compass, swab a deck, or steer a straight course. They indicate whether or not the person gets seasick.

> The voyage was unusually rough, but the General and Jesse proved themselves good sailors. Mrs. Grant suffered somewhat from sea-sickness, but, on the whole, enjoyed the voyage. . . . The General and Jesse never missed a meal, and the former smoked constantly—an excellent test of his sea-going abilities.
> —MCCABE, *A TOUR AROUND THE WORLD BY GENERAL GRANT*, 1879

Other expressions have been lost in the fog of time:

- **feeding Mother Carey's chickens**—Mother Carey's chickens are storm petrels, a common sea bird. This expression is a variant on "feeding the fish."

- **to know what wood the ship was made of**—The origin of this phrase is clear: sufferers spend a lot of time leaning over the rail, intently studying the side of the vessel.

> Philatus not accustomed to these narrow Seas, was more redy to tell what wood the ship was made of, than to aunswer to Euphues discourse.
> —JOHN LYLY, *EUPHUES AND HIS ENGLAND*, 1580

> It was no boote to bid him tell what the ship was made of, for he did it devoutly.
> —ROBERT ARMIN, *NEST OF NINNIES*, 1608

■ **puke**—The slang word *puke* has been around for a long
time. According to the Oxford English Dictionary its ori-
gins are uncertain, but probably trace to the late sixteenth
century, derived as an imitative form of the Late German
spucken, to spew or spit. The first written use in English occurs in 1600, in Shakespeare's *As You Like It*:

> . . . *the Infant, Mewling, and puking in the Nurses armes.*

Great poets have not been above using it when in search of an
appropriate rhyme:

> *There's not a sea the passenger e'er pukes in*
> *Turns up more dangerous breakers than the Euxine.*
> —LORD BYRON, *DON JUAN*, CIRCA 1820

In the Pacific Northwest of the United States, puker is the accepted slang term for a charter fishing boat.

> *They come, the cream and flow'r of all the Scots,*
> *   The children of politeness, science, wit,*
> *Exulting in their bench'd and gaudy boats,*
> *   Wherein some joking and some puking sit.*
> —WILLIAM TENNANT, *ANSTER FAIR*, 1812

■ **cascading**

> *I expected to have been caskading by this time, as some of our*
> *technical people have called it, i.e. vomiting.*
> —*JOURNAL OF THOMAS LARKIN TURNER*, 1832,
> MYSTIC SEAPORT MUSEUM

■ **cast up your accounts**

> *All day we have been pitching and rolling, producing a visible*
> *and rather "thinning" effect on our dinner table. I ate no sup-*
> *per, notwithstanding which precaution, I was obliged to "cast*
> *up my accounts" about half past nine.*
> —*JOURNAL OF CHARLES WHITE WATSON*, 1859,
> MYSTIC SEAPORT MUSEUM

And if you want to get your mind off your stomach with a game of cards, what better deck to reach for than this one (pūke is Chinese for playing cards. Really.):

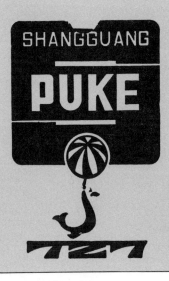

CHAPTER 9

Historical Perspective from the Rail

Don't feel too sorry for yourself the next time you're hanging over the rail. Your offering to the deep is part of a storied ritual that has played an important role in the course of human affairs.

Mal de mer is more than just another tuna fish sandwich tossed into a rolling sea; it has affected virtually every facet of life. Before modern air travel became a way of life there were no options for people who needed or wanted to cross bodies of water. If you chose not to travel by boat you chose not to travel at all.

Many people made that choice, creating an invisible barrier of fear—sort of a Great Wall of Chunder—that limited the exchange of people and ideas.

> *In nearly all the letters that I receive from my scientific friends in Europe the invitations to visit us in America are met with the statement that nothing prevents them but the dread of seasickness, of which they have some mild suggestions crossing the channel. Undoubtedly ten times as many Europeans would visit this country as now do, were it not for this fear.*
> —GEORGE M. BEARD, *A PRACTICAL TREATISE ON SEA-SICKNESS*, 1880

The Great Wall was a cultural and artistic barrier.

> *Lucien Guitry, France's greatest tragedian since Sully, obsti-*
> *nately declined all offers [to come to America] because he was*
> *sure that if he embarked he would be seasick and that if he*
> *was seasick he would die.*
> —BASIL WOON, *THE FRANTIC ATLANTIC,* 1927

European emigrants chose to travel out of economic, political, or religious necessity. Seasickness was just one of many hurdles they faced before starting a new life in America. In an early, semi-autobiographical novel Herman (*Moby Dick*) Melville wrote of the hardship of an Atlantic crossing:

> *. . . from the two "booby-hatches" came the steady hum of a*
> *subterranean wailing and weeping. That irresistible wrestler,*
> *sea-sickness, had overthrown the stoutest of their number, and*
> *the women and children were embracing and sobbing in all*
> *the agonies of the poor emigrant's first storm at sea.*
> —*REDBURN: HIS FIRST VOYAGE,* 1848

In at least one case, the choice *not* to travel proved to be a fatal mistake. In his rise to power the mad Roman emperor Caligula eliminated anyone and everyone who stood in his way. Caligula took advantage of a relative's fear of seasickness to bring about his downfall.

> *He had his brother Tiberius put to death without warning . . .*
> *and drove his father-in-law Silanus to end his life by cutting*
> *his throat with a razor. His charge against the latter was that*
> *Silanus had not followed him when he put to sea in stormy*
> *weather, but had remained behind in the hope of taking pos-*
> *session of the city in case he should be lost in the storm. . . .*
> *Now as a matter of fact, Silanus was subject to seasickness*
> *and wished to avoid the discomforts of the voyage . . .*
> —SUETONIUS, *LIFE OF CALIGULA,*
> 2ND CENTURY AD (ROLFE TRANSLATION, 1914)

If only Silanus had just been willing to hang over the rail for a while.

A willingness to accept the risk of being seasick proved politically advantageous in more recent times. In March 1950 President Harry S Truman made an ocean voyage from Washington, D.C., to Key West, Florida, on board the presidential yacht *Williamsburg*, a converted landing craft notorious for its wild motions. Bad weather had been forecast, and Truman could have chosen another form of travel. He went ahead with the trip anyway and, to the amusement of reporters trailing on a much larger, steadier vessel, got seasick. One writer saw tremendous political value in this:

> *He has forged another link with the masses. . . . The President invited the common lot of landlubbers afloat when he had every opportunity to avoid it. . . . He had promised the officers and crew of the yacht that he would take a voyage in her and had agreed that this was to be the occasion. Displaying, therefore, that trait which appears to mark a difference between Democrats and Republicans, and must account for a lot of votes, the President gave first consideration to the feelings of the sailors and declined to abandon the ship in which they take such pride.*
>
> *. . . the President did make the promise; he was warned not to keep it; he did keep it; he got as seasick on his yacht as the poor man in his hired boat; and thus he gave additional support to the thesis that Democrats act more humanly in public than Republicans, or at any rate have the luck to appear to do so.*
>
> *— THE NEW YORK TIMES, 1950*

One woman's experience with seasickness was elevated to the lofty environs of mythology. According to the ancient story of Jason and the Argonauts, the god Hermes sent a ram with a golden fleece to rescue Phrixus and his sister Helle from their wicked stepmother. During the escape Helle fell off the ram and drowned. The body of water was named the Hellespont (now called the Dardanelles, in Turkey) in her honor.

That's the way the story goes, but is it the way it really happened? Around 50 BC Diodorus of Sicily wrote an extensive *Library of History* of the known world, in which he discussed the truth behind some of the myths that were old even in his day. Diodorus had this to say about the escape:

> Many say that the true story is that Phrixus made his voyage on a ship which had the figurehead of a ram. They also say that Helle was suffering from seasickness and fell overboard when she accidentally leaned too far over the rail.

While some cross seas for pleasure, health, commerce, or an escape to a new life, others cross them for conquest. Troops are often moved by sea, and smart military planners allow for the effects of seasickness. In 47 BC Caesar sent a convoy of ships to Africa with the 13th and 14th legions, 800 Gallic cavalry, and 1,000 slingers and archers.

> With the wind behind them these ships arrived safely three days later. . . . He ordered his legions and cavalry to disembark and get over the effects of their lassitude and seasickness.
> —BELLUM AFRICANUM (WAY TRANSLATION, 1955)

Much of the modern research on seasick preventives has been motivated by military needs. One World War II general reportedly said that D-Day had resulted in the greatest mass vomiting in the history of mankind.

The history of science has also been influenced by seasickness. Charles Darwin was plagued by it during his famous five-year voyage on the *Beagle*. In his account, Darwin advised those who might think of imitating his adventure:

> If a person suffers much from sea-sickness, let him weigh it heavily in the balance. I speak from experience: it is no trifling evil, cured in a week.
> —CHARLES DARWIN, VOYAGE OF THE BEAGLE, 1839

If Darwin hadn't been seasick, he might not have spent so many days ashore, and evolutionary biology would never have been the same.

Seasickness has also made at least one inroad, albeit a failed one, into jurisprudence. One creative person invoked his suffering as a legal defense. The judge, obviously a landlubber, had little sympathy.

Seasickness Plea Fails

Seasickness is no excuse for failure to declare articles brought across the Channel upon which duty should be paid. The customs court of Dover has so held in the case of an Englishman coming from Ostend who failed to declare a gold watch, a revolver, opera glasses, and other things purchased in Belgium.

Notwithstanding the fact that the plea was entered that the man was so ill he was unable to list the articles the court imposed a fine of about $2,000.

— *The New York Times*, 1925

Seasickness has even been employed as a weapon by an over-enterprising journalist trying to get a scoop on aviation hero Charles Lindbergh. After his solo flight across the Atlantic in 1927 Lindbergh became an instant celebrity, and reporters hounded his every step. On May 27, 1929 he secretly married Anne Morrow, daughter of the United States ambassador to Mexico. The two slipped away from the family's Long Island estate for a quiet honeymoon cruise to Maine on their boat *Mouette*. Members of the media quickly picked up the trail:

> At one point I had to drag anchor to get away from a reporter in a launch who circled our boat repeatedly, hoping to bring us topside out of seasickness. But we managed to escape and enjoy our anonymity on the open water.
>
> — CHARLES LINDBERGH, *AUTOBIOGRAPHY OF VALUES*, 1976

The growth of the labor movement in the early 1900s aside, employers could still place unusual restrictions on some potential workers. For those thespians who might have wanted to pursue their work on the water, immunity to seasickness became a job requirement. In a 1907 article about a proposal to start staging plays on transatlantic steamers, *The New York Times* reported that "the actors and actresses engaged for the ocean theatre must carry certificates stating that they are proof against seasickness."

Such strictures no doubt prompted the empathy of fellow sufferers. Victims have to sympathize with one another since no one else will, and *mal de mer* may be one of the first illnesses to have had its own support group. The Anti-Seasickness League

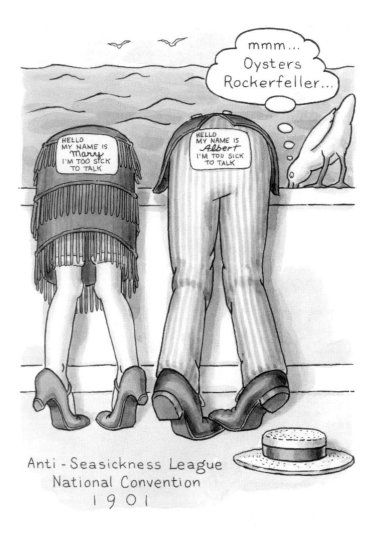

existed around 1900, based at 82 Boulevard Port-Royal, Paris. The group had its own publication, the *Journal de Mal de Mer et de la Santé à bord des Navires* (Journal of Seasickness and Health aboard Ships), which contained news on the disease and of ways to avoid it. The League participated in the European Health Exhibition at Ostend, Belgium, in 1901, although their display booth was not appreciated by all:

> *Its exhibits consist of nostrums, bandages, and various inge- nious devices which are supposed to set up conditions antago- nistic to those which produce seasickness; but the influence upon the visitor who examines them is said to be even worse than that due to the choppy seas of the Channel, since they recall very disagreeable memories and cause him to feel that his hold upon the kindly fruits of the earth and other comesti- bles he has assimilated is, at best, extremely tenuous.*
>
> —*THE NEW YORK TIMES,* 1901

CHAPTER 10

IT'S NOT EASY BEING GREEN
Serious Answers to Your
Seasickness Questions

Science may eventually conquer seasickness, but until then you'll have to avoid it or endure it. Knowing what causes seasickness—sensory conflict—you can take simple steps to minimize the chances of being afflicted, regardless of the boat's size. Modern cruise ships provide a steady ride in almost all sea conditions, and modern medicine offers a variety of clinically tested preventives. Here's some advice based on the latest information about *mal de mer* and how to avoid it.

Will I become seasick?

Studies have shown that if you are healthy there is about a 90 percent chance that you can become seasick if conditions are right and you haven't taken steps to prevent it. Sailors even have a saying: "If you've never been seasick, you just haven't sailed enough."

Individuals differ in their inherent susceptibility, which can be broken down into two areas:

Receptivity. Your sensitivity to the changed motions at sea. If your receptivity is high, small motions could overcome you quickly. If it's low, it could take a long time for even extremely rough weather to have an effect.

Adaptability. How quickly you adapt to the changed motions at sea – getting your sea legs. The faster you adapt to the constant motion, the sooner you'll be free of the ailment, no matter how rough it gets.

Only a very few people have constitutions that will allow them to get sick and stay sick, and even they can be helped by modern remedies.

There does tend to be a variation in susceptibility with age, as we showed in Chapter 1, but recent studies have shown that the old belief that women are more susceptible than men is just a myth.

Does it matter what type of boat or ship I go out in?

Yes. Every vessel has its own characteristic responses to the sea's motions. Larger ships are more stable in general, but there can be wide individual differences. Many modern ships, especially cruise ships, which have a high incidence of first-time sailors, have active or passive anti-roll mechanisms that have virtually banished seasickness aboard.

What medicines can I take to prevent seasickness?

There is a great deal of effective medication available, both prescription and over-the-counter. Unfortunately, no single drug works well for everyone, so you must find which is right for you. Try some of the non-prescription drugs, like Dramamine, Bonine, or Marezine. If these don't do the trick see your family physician or the ship's doctor. Many people have had good luck with Transderm-Scop, small patches worn behind the ears that release scopolamine into your system over a period of days.

Almost all of the medications take some time to get into your system and start working, so if you take them when you start feeling queasy, it's too late. One of the real benefits of anti-seasickness drugs is that they raise your threshold of vulnerability. This allows you to stay active longer without getting sick, during which time you become adapted and no longer need the drugs. Some of these medicines can have side effects, so it is always a good idea to consult a doctor, and try them on land before the trip to see if they affect you in any way.

Useful Anti-Motion Sickness Drugs

Generic Name/ Brand Name	Mfr.	Form	OTC/Rx	Duration Of Action
Dimenhydrinate				
Dramamine	Seale	50 mg tablet;	OTC	4–6 hr
		liquid	OTC	4–6 hr
		50 mg injection	Rx	4–6 hr
Dramamine	Richardson-Vicks	50 mg chewable tab	OTC	4–6 hr
Gravol	Homer	75 mg timed-release capsule;	OTC (B&C)	6 hr
		suppository	OTC (B&C)	6 hr
Meclizine HCl				
Bonine	Leeming	25 mg chewable tab	OTC	6–12 hr
Antivert	Roerig	12.5; 25; 50 mg tab	Rx	6–12 hr
Meclizine	Geneva	12.5 mg tab	OTC	6–12 hr
Cinnarizine				
Stugeron	Janssen	15 mg tab	Rx (UK&B)	6–12 hr
Cyclizin				
Marezine	Burroughs	50 mg capsule;	OTC	4–6 hr
		injection	Rx	4–6 hr
Scopolamine HBR				
Kwells	Nicholas	0.3 mg tablet	OTC (UK&B)	4–6 hr
Transdermal Scopolamine				
Transderm-Scop	CIBA	1.5 mg skin patch	Rx,OTC (B&C)	2–3 days

(table continued)

Generic Name/ Brand Name	Mfr.	Form	OTC/Rx	Duration Of Action
Scopolamine HBR & Dextroamphetamine				
Scopolamine + Dexedrine	SKF	03. mg scop + 5.0 mg dex tabs tablets	Rx	4–6 hr
Promethazine				
Phenergan	Wyeth	12.5; 25; 50 mg tab;	Rx	6–12 hr
		suppository;	Rx	6–12 hr
		injection	Rx	6–12 hr
Promethazine & Ephedrine				
Phenergan +	Wyeth	25 mg phenergan +		
Ephedrine		25 mg ephe-drine (tablets)	Rx	6–12 hr

OTC = over the counter **Rx** = by prescription only **OTC (B&C)** = OTC in Bermuda & Canada **OTC (UK&B)** = OTC in UK & Bermuda

(Charles Oman, courtesy of Cruising World)

Will the remedies in Chapter 3 work?

Almost all of the preventives and cures in Chapter 3 work by the placebo effect (see Tinkerbell cures), if they work at all. As Abraham Lincoln might have said, the problem with placebos is that they seem to help only a small number of people, and those people only some of the time. Rather than spending money on the latest motion-sickness miracle cure, you're better off finding a scientifically tested medication that works for you.

What can I eat or drink to prevent seasickness?

There really is no scientific evidence that consuming one thing or another makes any difference. So enjoy—in moderation—those delicious, hearty meals traditionally served at sea, and don't eat things that would make you sick on shore. Stay away from alcoholic beverages, despite all the traditional references to it in Chapter 3. Alcohol affects inner ear function, and will just make you sicker.

What shipboard activities help prevent seasickness?

Lying down may make you feel better temporarily, but it doesn't do much to help you adapt. The more you move around, the sooner you'll become accustomed to the boat's motions. Don't try to do anything that requires a close visual focus, like reading, navigating, or splicing a line. If you have to carry out a task that could make you seasick, try to take breaks at frequent intervals. Be sure you have a broad view of the waves and the horizon, and try to anticipate the vessel's motions. If you're on a small boat, ask to take a turn at the helm.

Where on the ship am I least likely to get seasick?

On any kind of vessel, find a dry, safe spot with plenty of fresh air and a clear view of the horizon. A boat's motions are least pronounced at its center, so avoid the extreme bow or stern, and stay away from the rail.

Where on the ship am I most likely to get seasick?

In any enclosed space with no broad view of the horizon. On a small boat this is belowdecks, but on a large vessel this could be your cabin on an upper deck. This is where sensory conflict is the greatest; everything looks stable, but your vestibular system and muscles can sense the motion. If you must go inside, keep your visits short.

Where should I go to be seasick?

"The rail" is the popular answer but usually not the right one. Being near the side of a ship in rough weather can be dangerous even if you're feeling well and alert, and is even more so if you're seasick. On a large vessel it's safer to use a bathroom—or even vomit on deck if you just can't wait. It's easier to clean up a mess than to pull someone out of the water. On a small vessel, wear a safety harness and clip it to something solid.

How should you treat a serious case of seasickness?

Seasickness can become a serious medical condition if vomiting continues over a long period, with the sufferer becoming dangerously weakened and dehydrated. It is important to take some food and liquids, even if they don't stay down very long. If there is medical help aboard, take advantage of it. If necessary, cut the trip short and get the patient ashore.

Just when you thought it was safe to get off the water . . .

Congratulations! You've braved the high seas, and though you might have gotten seasick at the outset, you're now fully adapted—an old salt. But your problems may not be over. After a voyage, sailors have been known to step ashore and become violently ill. This is known as *mal de débarquement* (going-ashore sickness). Your brain now expects constant motion as the normal condition, and may perceive the stability of shore as abnormal.

Bon Voyage!

Xmas gift
mier Ka metcafe
midland, mi
1992